Tai Chi
for health
& vitality

A comprehensive guide to the short yang form

Robert Parry

hamlyn

First published in Great Britain in 2005 by
Hamlyn, a division of Octopus Publishing Ltd
2–4 Heron Quays, London E14 4JP

Distributed in the United States and Canada by
Sterling Publishing Co., Inc.
387 Park Avenue South,
New York, NY 10016–8810

ISBN 0 600 61090 X
EAN 9780600610908

A CIP catalgue record for this book is available
from the British Library

Printed and bound in China

10 9 8 7 6 5 4 3 2 1

Tai chi is a safe, gentle exercise and an excellent
means of staying fit and well. However, please
remember that tai chi cannot be used for the treatment
of illness, nor is it a cure for serious disease. The
author and publisher cannot accept responsibility for
any misadventure resulting from inappropriate use of
the techniques outlined in this book. Always seek
professional medical advice before undertaking any
new exercise programme.

Contents

Introduction

Tiger and Golden Pheasant, Crane Bird and Snake, Cloudy Hands and Monkey! These are some of the images named in the sequence of slow, graceful movement known as tai chi. Health, vitality, moving meditation and vital energy weave their paths through the lives of those who practise tai chi. This is the magic that underlies the gentle art: 'breathing made visible' – the essence of tai chi as it appears in this book.

When I first began teaching and writing about tai chi in the early 1990s, things were different. You would have to explain very carefully what tai chi was – that special, mysterious exercise from China. You would have to extol the benefits of tai chi in terms of health in order to convince people that it was relaxing, calming and, at the same time, strangely energizing! But things have changed. Most of us now have some notion of what tai chi is and how it looks. At the very least, we have all seen glimpses of it in films, on television or during our vacations or travels to the East. Most big-city parks now have tai chi enthusiasts strutting their stuff in the early mornings, and clubs and classes are springing up everywhere. Because of this, many people are now starting to feel that there is something worth investigating in these graceful, dance-like movements.

Of course, being aware of something is very different to actually taking part. There are still plenty of spectators out there, people on the sidelines who are attracted to tai chi's unique qualities and special elegance, but who remain uncertain as to how to get started. They would love to give it a try, but it's a matter of time, or of confidence, of getting to know where to go and who to ask. I can understand this, because I once felt that way myself. It was only by stumbling upon a small class of pioneer tai chi enthusiasts in my neighbourhood that I got the break and started to learn.

So, do not worry if you have never tried tai chi before. Follow the instructions in these pages and you will almost certainly come away with a sense of how tai chi feels.

When you begin to practise tai chi, you will discover how it can:
• improve your sense of balance
• increase your self-confidence
• improve your general fitness
• help to boost your resistance to common illnesses such as colds or flu

In time, you might even be able to use tai chi to control stress, to relax more and to locate that much-sought-after 'inner peace' which, in this noisy and chaotic world, we all sometimes wish we could reach out to and grab for ourselves. Sounds good? Well, *it is good!*

If you are aiming to look after yourself with some gentle, inspiring exercise, you need look no further than tai chi. If you are seeking a means of controlling stress, here it is. If you are curious about the ideas and beliefs of other cultures, tai chi is a great way of beginning to explore and to understand.

TAI CHI FOR ALL

So, who is tai chi for? What sort of people? The answer is: just about everybody! Tai chi is suitable for all ages and all levels of fitness. Whether you are a super-athlete or a couch potato, young or old, you can gain something from practising these wonderful, graceful movements. Tai chi can be enjoyed by the able-bodied and the disabled, and even to a certain extent while seated.

No one is barred entry to the world of tai chi – although the one thing you will need is a degree of dedication, since it takes a while (usually months rather than weeks) to learn the whole sequence of movements and to feel comfortable doing them. Once you can go all the way through the sequence from start to finish, however, the real magic begins and all manner of positive changes can take place within you.

Gentle, invigorating, early-morning exercise is a way of life in China.

BENEFITS

Ultimately, the tai chi experience varies for different people, but it usually enhances your abilities in whatever field you are active.

- For artists and dancers, there is improved performance and creativity.
- For salesmen, there is greater confidence.
- For therapists, there is increased rapport with their patients.
- For those recovering from illness, there is speedier rehabilitation.
- For golfers, there is a better swing.

Whatever sphere you move in, you will find that tai chi can open new doorways to new experiences, helping you make the most of what you do.

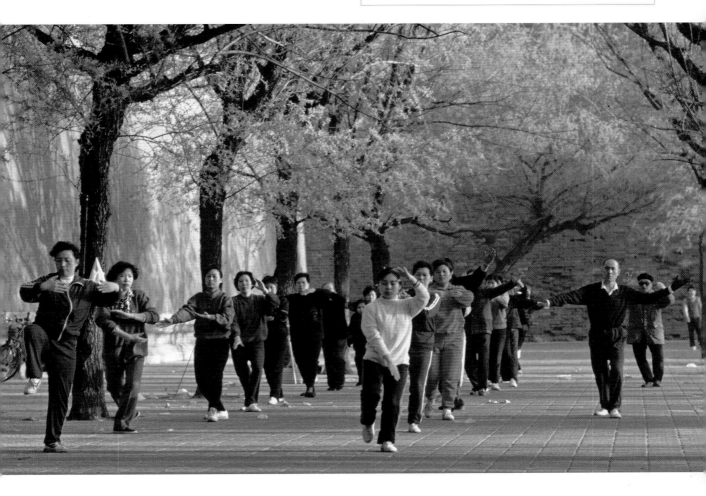

Put another way: tai chi helps us to sit more comfortably within ourselves, and that can be a really good feeling.

Why 'tai chi'?

The Chinese word *tai* means 'great', while *chi* can be variously translated as 'ultimate' or – especially in popular usage – 'energy'. It's all about ultimate energy, therefore, a kind of cultivation of life force through exercise. Chi is everywhere, in all things. It is what sustains us in all our endeavours. It helps us to move, and it helps us to breathe. It helps us to resist disease, and also to think and to make decisions. It is alive as much in our thoughts as in our bones. Put another way: tai chi helps us to sit more comfortably within ourselves, and that can be a really good feeling.

Yet even this does not adequately describe the full extent of tai chi's range and influence. Many people will remind you that tai chi is also a martial art, especially when studied at its highest levels. The martial arts flourished in China during the 12th and 13th centuries, when people blended the techniques of combat and traditions of therapeutic exercise into what is known as Tai Chi Ch'uan. That is why the movements have a strong, dynamic quality, even when they are used as a means of relaxation. However, no amount of written instructions can ever train you in the skills required to use tai chi as a martial art, and I would certainly not be able to teach you.

RELAXATION THROUGH EXERCISE

As a practitioner of oriental medicine, I have always been excited by the advantages that tai chi brings to people in terms of health and fitness, and so the tai chi presented here is concerned solely with these objectives. It is also the kind of tai chi sometimes referred to as a 'moving meditation'. There is nothing

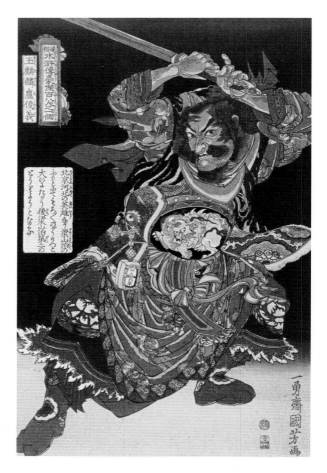

Tai chi origins lie in the martial traditions of the East.

particularly weird or mystical about this. 'Moving meditation' simply means that tai chi can help you reach a state of inner calm, while at the same time providing plenty of interest and activity for the physical body. It therefore remains always practical, always rooted in reality. Tai chi encourages you to relax without becoming bored.

Relaxation is a strange thing. We know the word, but many of us will never really have experienced how it feels. When asked, for example, 'What sort of things do you do to relax?', people will answer, 'Oh, I go to the cinema', or 'I'm into basketball', or 'I just like to chill out with the family and kids'. In practice, none of these activities is in the least bit relaxing. They may be fun, and perhaps a good way of letting off steam, but they usually just involve additional stresses for the body and the mind. Relaxation, as we will be using the word in tai chi, means being able to let go of tension – to leave behind, even if only for 10 minutes a day, the endless treadmill of stress, competition, stimulation, and emotional ups and downs that most recreational activities demand. We do this, however, not by turning off from our body, but by working with it. We do it with exercise, but exercise that is calming as well as rooted in the real world.

THE MIDDLE WAY

I believe that this sense of realism – of having your feet planted firmly on the ground – is an important aspect of tai chi, because no matter what our personal goals might be in studying any kind of relaxation technique, we all need to maintain a certain level of stamina and mental clarity if we are to function successfully in the real world. The qualities of balance and inner strength that are clearly observed whenever you see the art being demonstrated by a master, are ones for which even the most humble of tai chi enthusiasts should strive, no matter how imperfectly. If you can use tai chi in this way, blending the practical with the inspirational, you will come to experience a real sense of achievement and self-confidence that will reach out to colour every aspect of your life, at work and at play.

Ultimately, therefore, tai chi is all about finding what the scholars of ancient China called the Middle Way – the 'sweet spot' between being a physical body and a thinking, feeling individual. And although everyone may have their own notion about what that Middle Way might be, taking the first steps on that special journey of discovery is, I like to think, what this book is all about. I hope you will agree and that you will enjoy what comes next.

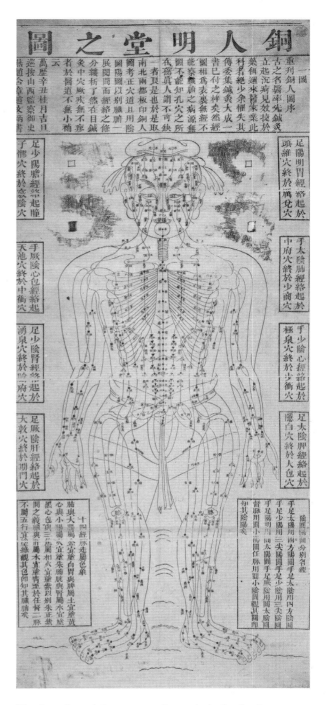

The location of the energy channels in the body was mapped out long ago in ancient China.

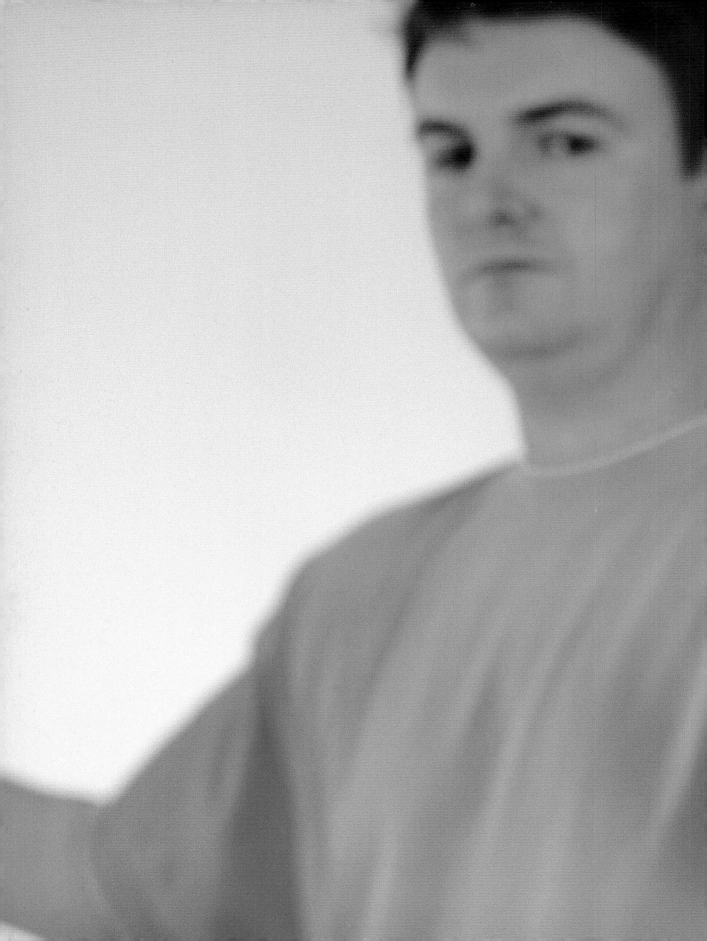

what is
tai chi?

The Short Yang Form

You could say that tai chi is 'breathing made visible' – a combination of slow-moving exercise combined with calm, regular breathing. It is the rhythm and pace of the breath that shapes the speed at which the movements themselves are enacted. This is different to most other forms of exercise, in which the breath simply follows the movements, sometimes in a rather haphazard fashion.

The other important feature of tai chi is that it is based on a precise sequence of movements, usually handed down through the generations, and that sequence does not alter: the movements are always performed in the same order. This sequence is called a 'form'. There are many different tai chi forms in the world today, reflecting different tai chi styles and traditions – even within each style, there can be several variations. The form on which we will concentrate in this book is one of the most popular, called the Short Yang Form.

Incidentally, the word 'Yang' as used in this context has nothing to do with Yin and Yang, which are explained on pages 16–17. Yang is simply the name of the family who originated the style: the Yang style of tai chi. The Short Form was created by one of the Yang family's pupils, Cheng Man Ch'ing, who lived from 1900 to 1975. Cheng Man Ch'ing was not only a great teacher of tai chi, but also a practitioner of herbal medicine, a professor of literature, a painter and a calligrapher. If any one person can be credited with helping tai chi to become popular and accepted outside its native China during the last century, it is Cheng Man Ch'ing, and his form remains as a great and lasting testimony to his skill in communicating the essence of such a complex art to so many people. He developed the Short Yang Form to promote tai chi's health-giving properties, and to make it relatively easy for westerners to learn compared to some of the more traditional and martial-oriented forms. So it is ideal for our purposes.

A typical forward-stepping sequence of tai chi.

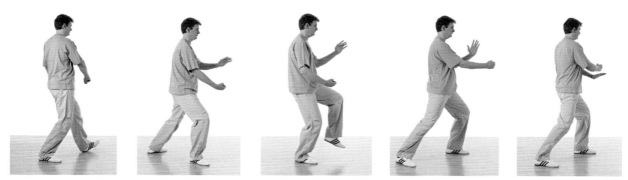

Principles of Tai Chi

We will be looking closely at the physical characteristics of tai chi exercise in detail in the next chapter and beyond, where each movement is explained in step-by-step detail. But first of all, how does it all work, and moreover, what is so special about daily tai chi practice that it can bestow all these wonderful health-giving qualities?

To answer these questions, we have to go back in time and look at the cultures from which exercises of this kind first arose. Although the tai chi that we enjoy today has its beginning around the 13th century AD, even then it was closely related to the philosophy and medical practices of Chinese culture thousands of years earlier. This is where we have to look, way back in the distant past, to locate the true origins of tai chi.

The most important principle, and the one big idea you need to take on board when seeking an explanation of how tai chi (or, indeed, oriental medicine) works, is the existence of a universal energy or life force. This, as we have already seen, is called 'chi' – sometimes written as Qi – and it flows through all things in nature, from the tiniest microbe to the greatest star.

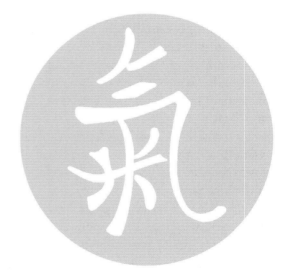

The Chinese character for chi (or Qi).

KEY FEATURES OF TAI CHI

- Slow, gentle, non-tensile movement.
- Calm, regular breathing.
- Assists muscle tone.
- Assists circulation.
- Stimulates the lymphatic system.

- Strengthens immunity to common ailments.
- Promotes relaxation.
- Encourages mental clarity, creativity and self-confidence.
- Develops inner calm.

The Jingluo

In the human body, the chi flows through what is considered to be a collection of channels, also known as meridians. These were mapped out thousands of years ago by the brilliant physicians of ancient China and they are still referred to and used today in clinical practice by thousands of acupuncturists, masseurs, herbalists and healers all over the world.

Some of these channels are large, and flow through the major organs of the body, from which they derive their names. So, for example, we have the Liver channel, which originates in the toes and then flows up the body through the liver itself, finishing in the chest. There is a Bladder channel, running along the back, and a Lung channel that flows from the chest through the arms to the thumbs – altogether, there are 14 major channels. There are also numerous minor channels and many more even smaller, capillary-like ones, all of which help to circulate the chi around the body. The collective name for all the channel pathways is the Jingluo, and through this special medium all the cells, bones, muscles and sinews are constantly fed and stimulated by life-giving energy.

The movements of tai chi are thought to enhance and expedite the journey of chi through the Jingluo. Certain movements stimulate certain channels in a subtle way, as we shall see. You don't have to know about any of this to reap the benefits of the exercises, but sometimes you may actually feel the energy flowing along your limbs or around your body as you progress through the tai chi sequence – this is the chi moving strongly, nourishing all the organs and systems of the body along the way. It is simply a further confirmation of the efficacy of this wonderful system of exercise.

THE VITAL CENTRE

There are also key areas in the body where chi is concentrated and stored. Tai chi, and related disciplines such as chi kung and yoga, teach us that these are located in places such as the lower abdomen, the chest and the small of the back between the kidneys. In tai chi we endeavour to be mindful of these places, and in particular the one called the Tan Tien (also sometimes written as Dan Dien), which is situated just beneath the navel. It is also commonly known as the 'vital centre' of the body.

Most, if not all, of the tai chi movements are directed from this place. The constant rotation of the waist and accompanying stimulation of this vital centre in tai chi exercise helps in the generation and release of what is called 'internal energy'. This is then projected into the limbs, and in particular the hands and feet, as you work. Some people experience this as a tingling, others as a cool energy, others (paradoxically) as heat. Some never feel it at all, but this does not matter.

If you are already engaged in holistic therapies such as massage, shiatsu, aromatherapy or any other hands-on medical treatment, you will be aware of how helpful it can be to establish a link, even if only on a mental level, between the vital centre of the body and your hands.

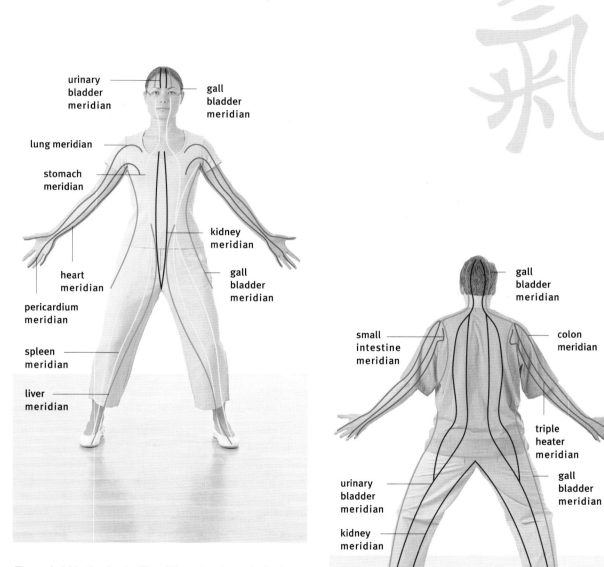

urinary
bladder
meridian

gall
bladder
meridian

lung meridian

stomach
meridian

kidney
meridian

heart
meridian

gall
bladder
meridian

pericardium
meridian

spleen
meridian

liver
meridian

gall
bladder
meridian

small
intestine
meridian

colon
meridian

triple
heater
meridian

gall
bladder
meridian

urinary
bladder
meridian

kidney
meridian

*Flow of chi in the body. The different colours indicate
the various organs through which the energy flows.
Green shows the channels of the Liver and Gall
Bladder, Blue the Kidneys and Bladder, and so on.*

Yang and Yin

The second important principle underlying the movement of chi within the body also traces its origin back to the ancient cultures and medical philosophies of the East. This is the celebrated pairing of Yang and Yin. One of the ways the chi is able to move through the body is via the interplay of these two great polarities, which are considered to be at work within all of nature.

Viewed as a kind of positive/negative dynamism, Yang and Yin are usually considered to be opposites, but they do also have a mutually supporting relationship and can even change from one into the other. A glance at the table should help to clarify the nature of these two great, alternating phases of energy.

All of these opposites are interdependent, always subject to change. Collectively, they have come to be represented by a universal concept that is actually called the 'Tai Chi'. This state of oneness is mentioned in the ancient classic of Chinese literature the *I Ching* or *Book of Changes*, parts of which date back to the

YANG	YIN
Light	Dark
Day	Night
Summer	Winter
Spring	Autumn
Dry	Moist
Warm	Cool
Fiery	Watery
Active	Passive
Expansion	Contraction
Forward	Reverse
Spirit	Matter
Activity	Stillness
Forthright	Reserved
Firm	Yielding

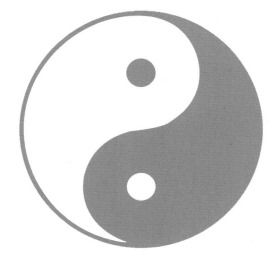

12th century BC. Later, all this came to be encapsulated in the famous symbol known as the tai chi tu, the popular diagram illustrated here that we all recognize today. You can see how the circle or sphere is divided into light and dark by a gently curving line, suggesting movement and change, while the two small points, one situated within each half, represent the seeds or latent potential for change always present at the heart of each polarity. So Summer (Yang), for instance, is always ready to change into Winter (Yin), Light into Dark, Day into Night, and vice versa.

YIN AND YANG IN TAI CHI

In the tai chi form, too, each of the movements has a Yin and a Yang aspect to it. To begin, there is usually a gathering-in, preparatory position (Yin), followed by a forward, outward-thrusting movement (Yang). Then the whole cycle begins again with the next gathering-in position. This Yin-into-Yang interplay continues throughout the sequence in a calm, regular fashion and is assisted by the movement of the breath. We tend to match the Yin phase of each movement to our inhalation, and then, a moment later, match the Yang phase to our exhalation.

The breath dictates the pace at which Yin changes to Yang and each movement changes into the other. This constant dynamic interchange helps us to transport the chi within the body and has enormous benefits in terms of health. Wherever the chi is able to move efficiently through the Jingluo, the body is alive and supple; where chi is absent, however, stagnation and decay will usually set in. Movement and change are at the heart of all of life, therefore, and at the core of tai chi also.

Benefits of Tai Chi

So, what exactly are the benefits of tai chi, and how long will it take to experience all these positive changes? Well, bearing in mind that tai chi is never a substitute for medical treatment, and assuming you practise daily and are willing to devote at least 10–15 minutes to your session, you may begin to notice an improvement in your balance, flexibility and physical co-ordination within just a few weeks.

A lot depends on your starting point, of course, which includes your current state of health and your age. Those who are robust and strong will clearly have a head-start on those whose health is more frail. Even so, minor health problems should begin to become more manageable after a few months, as your overall vitality gradually begins to strengthen and your circulation and respiration improve through increased levels of fitness. There are, therefore, very clear benefits for the cardiovascular system – the heart and lungs – at an early stage.

In this book, where applicable, specific health benefits are listed alongside the relevant movements – those that exert particular influences on certain parts of the body, for example, or on certain internal organs. However, the benefits of tai chi in terms of health are perhaps more obvious in the overall cumulative effect of all the movements taken together over time. As the months go by, and you become more involved in your tai chi studies, you may also notice changes in your ability to manage stress and tension, and an increase in your self-confidence.

Wei Chi

Your resistance to common ailments such as colds and flu further improves as the immune function in your

> **BENEFITS**
>
> **With regular practice, tai chi:**
> - Provides gentle aerobic exercise.
> - Allows you to let go of physical tension.
> - Helps tone the muscles of the legs, waist and buttocks.
> - Strengthens immunity to common ailments.
> - Helps you to relax and stay calm.
> - Assists the functioning of the lymphatic system.
> - Helps the heart, lungs and digestive organs to perform more efficiently.
> - Promotes creativity and self-confidence.

body becomes more robust. Tai chi strengthens the immune system by boosting what is called the Wei Chi, which is the term used in oriental medicine for the body's defensive energy that helps us fight off infection. The Wei Chi is closely related to the function of the lungs. It is centred in the chest but spreads out all over the body to form a 'protective shield'.

The lymphatic system

To say that tai chi works because it promotes the flow of energy around the body is all well and good, but there are some additional explanations that have a more scientific basis. In particular, the slow, non-tensile movements of tai chi are enormously helpful in stimulating the lymphatic system of the body. We occasionally become aware of our lymph nodes at times of illness. Concentrated in specific areas such as the throat, chest, armpits, groin, elbows and knees, they swell and can become painful when illness threatens. This is because the lymphatic function is a major component of the immune system, working away silently to maintain a state of internal equilibrium at every moment and help rid the body of all the toxins and bacterial, viral and fungal infections that can make us unwell.

MOVEMENT WITHOUT TENSION

The important point here is that although the body has a means of transporting waste matter and toxins into the lymphatic system, the lymph fluid that performs this function does not have a pump – as the blood has the heart, for example – to circulate it around the body. Instead, it relies to a great extent on movement, on the body pushing and squeezing the process along by itself as it goes about its daily tasks.

The difficulty for us in today's stressful world is that it is precisely those areas of the body so vital to the efficient workings of the lymphatic system – chest, armpits, groin and so on – that are often so bound up with tension that this process becomes severely restricted. Even when we are active and exercising hard, these areas can remain tight and prone to congestion simply through muscular tension.

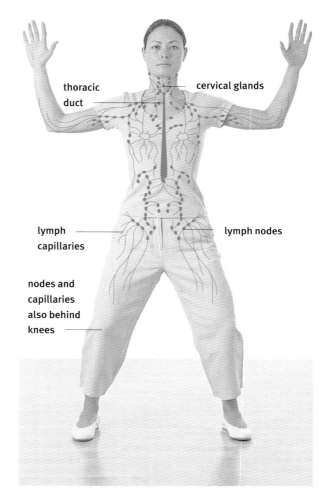

thoracic duct

cervical glands

lymph capillaries

lymph nodes

nodes and capillaries also behind knees

The body's lymph system helps to drain toxins from the body and combats infection.

Tai chi, on the other hand, with its open, gentle and non-tensile movements, provides an ideal stimulus for the lymphatic system. Movement without tension is therefore one of the main reasons why tai chi is so profoundly beneficial to our health. With daily practice, it aids the body's constant efforts to rid itself of damaging toxins and bacteria. In oriental medicine, all this corresponds once again to the concept of the Wei Chi: the body's 'protective shield'.

Stress management

Tai chi is particularly relevant in today's hectic world as a stress-busting tool. Stress has long been known as a contributory factor in numerous serious illnesses, so controlling our response to it is vital to our well-being and can act directly on the very source of so many of our most serious health hazards.

There are all sorts of ideas about how we can best deal with the pains and strains of modern living. There is even a view that stress is not always such a bad thing, because it is usually part and parcel of a stimulating, successful and fulfilling lifestyle. However, too much stress can become counter-productive, dominating our lives to the point of damaging our health and preventing us from enjoying the very things we have worked so hard to achieve.

Some people believe they can break this vicious cycle through recreational pursuits – competitive sports, watching violent movies, stressful journeys to exotic destinations, and so on – that, oddly enough, can be even more stressful than their daily lives. Much of this simply replaces one form of stress with another. Letting off steam, as it is called, has its place in stress management, but it does not reach to the root cause of the problem, which is our internal state. As we have seen, tai chi addresses that root cause by establishing a calm internal state.

USING TAI CHI TO COMBAT STRESS

Because it does not require any special preparation, clothing or location, tai chi can be incorporated into your daily stress-management routine very easily. You can start your day with it – a very popular choice in China, where tai chi is widely used – or you can wind down and finish your day with a little tai chi, as it helps to set you up for sleep. You can even fit a quick session into your lunch break or at any other point during the day.

Do not be fooled by the inner voice that says to you: 'Oh, today has been so awful and I am feeling so bad that nothing is going to make it better.' That is simply not true. It is the Inner Slouch speaking, a part of you that regularly proffers all manner of ingenious excuses for not doing something positive for yourself. Don't listen to it! Try tai chi instead. Do it, and you will feel different. Tai chi really is something you can turn to at any time for help.

ABDOMINAL BREATHING

Once you are familiar with the whole sequence and are able to shape it around your natural rhythm of breathing, without too much conscious effort, you can further enhance tai chi's relaxing qualities by incorporating what is called 'abdominal breathing'. In this, the abdomen is relaxed and expands at the commencement of the inhalation. It is as if we are 'breathing' into the tummy for a moment rather than the lungs, which are of course located much higher up in the chest. This allows the important muscle called the diaphragm (situated just below the lower ribs), to descend and so greatly assist the lungs in the taking in of air. This movement is very subtle, and should under no circumstances ever be forced or strained. Simply be aware of the tendency for the abdomen to expand with the inhalation, and eventually this style of breathing will start to occur all by itself. It is also an excellent way of aiding medititation and relaxation at any time, even if you are just seated in a chair.

'Fight or flight' versus rest

One way to understand tai chi's unique stress-busting properties is through the workings of the autonomic nervous system, which regulates our internal organs and controls heartbeat, digestion and so on. Although these activities cannot be influenced by our will, they are affected in a subtle way by our feelings and state of mind.

FIGHT OR FLIGHT

The system has two distinct modes of operation. The first is called the sympathetic mode, where the functions of the body related to the 'fight-or-flight' survival instinct are on high alert. Today, although we are continually activated and stressed into the fight-or-flight reaction, we are usually unable to give vent to it. Being stuck in a traffic jam, for instance, is all about fight or flight – making us alert and anxious, but with nowhere to run! The body can usually cope with this, and becomes calm in time. If it happens too often, however, the body can become locked into a state of permanent stress arousal, anxiety and nervous tension. Unable to relax at all, the entire physical and mental system gradually exhausts itself of energy and health.

RESTING PHASE

Fortunately, there is a second mode of functioning for the nervous system called the parasympathetic mode or resting phase. This kicks in at times of calm, when we are relaxed and feel safe and secure; it nourishes and replenishes our cells and allows us to rest and to sleep.

Tai chi enables you to switch into that gentle, nurturing, resting phase relatively easily, and can therefore exert an exceptionally positive effect in

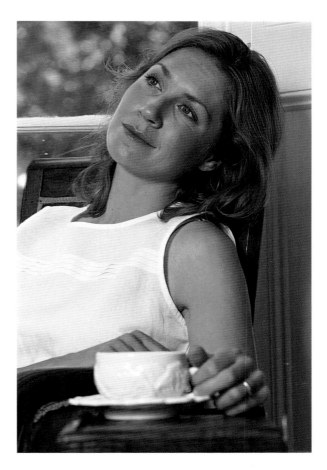

Everyone needs to take time out to combat stress.

terms of health. Any form of relaxation can achieve this switch, of course, but tai chi is especially suitable because it does not involve enforced stillness. This unique quality of tai chi, different to almost any other form of relaxation therapy, is that you can keep moving while you do it (the 'moving meditation' again, mentioned in our introduction) – and so the transition from 'fight or flight' to resting state is far easier than, say, forcing yourself to 'sit down and relax' – which is often very difficult to achieve anyway after a stressful day. So even from the perspective of western anatomy and physiology, there are lots of real issues that can be resolved through the practice of tai chi. Over time, it can really make a difference to how successfully we are able to integrate stress into our daily lives and so avoid the kinds of adverse physical reactions that stress can bring about.

Weight control

You may be wondering if tai chi will help you to become slimmer and more attractive. If you agree that those who are full of vitality and self-confidence are more attractive to others, then perhaps the answer is yes! But what about slimming?

The main concern of many people is that of being overweight, due in part to our modern, sedentary lifestyle and lack of suitable exercise. As you probably know, *any* form of exercise – including just moving around a little more in your daily life – is better than none and will help you to shed the pounds. However, the important key to using exercise successfully for weight control is that it has to be something you can engage in regularly, and this is difficult unless you enjoy what you are doing.

Tai chi is something you will enjoy, I hope, because it is interesting and constantly challenging – and so more likely to help you succeed in establishing a workable exercise programme. Rather than a swift once-a-week visit to the gym, or a bit of reluctant jogging in the evenings, tai chi is something you will be *looking forward* to doing each day. It provides that all-important foundation of regularity. Moreover, tai chi is also an ideal means of warming up or 'warming down' when you are involved in more strenuous exercises or sports.

Other effects

Tai chi can also aid slimmers in a more subtle way, because it naturally increases the body's intake of oxygen. Oxygen is needed to make things burn – and that includes calories. If you can get an efficient and generous oxygen supply to the cells of the body, this will serve to support you in the task of reducing fat and burning off excess energy.

Finally, we have seen how tai chi helps to stimulate the circulation of lymph fluid around the body. This is important, because poorly circulating lymph can lead to a build-up of fluid and fat beneath the skin, and the formation of cellulite. A well-functioning lymphatic system, on the other hand, together with the increased intake of oxygen that tai chi provides, assists in the maintenance of fresh, radiant skin through better cellular regeneration and the improved circulation of vital nutrients.

People spend a lot of time and money in the quest for good skin. Creams and ointments, pills and potions are useful, and have their part to play. But ultimately it is our inner health that is the most significant ingredient in maintaining a fresh, youthful appearance.

BENEFITS

In summary, tai chi can help with weight control by:

- Providing an exercise regime you can enjoy and stick to.
- Increasing the body's intake of oxygen and burning of calories.
- Stimulating the circulation of lymph fluid, thereby reducing the build-up of fat and cellulite.

Remember that daily practice is essential if you wish to derive any significant weight-control benefits.

Beyond the body

In quantifying the benefits of regular tai chi practice, there is also the internal dimension to consider – the effect that tai chi can have on your feelings and self-confidence. In fact, any form of exercise is likely to make you feel good, since it helps to release hormones in the brain called endorphins, which produce a gentle 'high' that lifts the spirit in a unique way.

However, the effects of tai chi on the inner state extend much further than that. Once you have learned the form and are practising regularly, you will begin to approach a very special space, called Wu Wei by scholars of ancient Chinese philosophy.

Wu Wei corresponds in part to the highly relaxed 'alpha state' of brain waves measured by western science – a condition which, if repeated regularly, leads to numerous positive changes in overall attitude and outlook on life. For example:

- You should begin to notice an increase in creative energy, with ideas coming more easily.
- Solutions to problems may present themselves more readily, perhaps because you can relax more and see the alternatives.
- You might also find that you are endowed with a greater sense of self-esteem and a little more optimism than before.

LETTING GO

All this works simply through the invaluable process of being able to 'let go'. The notion of becoming empty and letting go is not a negative state. Tai chi and the philosophy that attends it, called Taoism, urges us to 'let go' constantly. This is important. If we remain full to

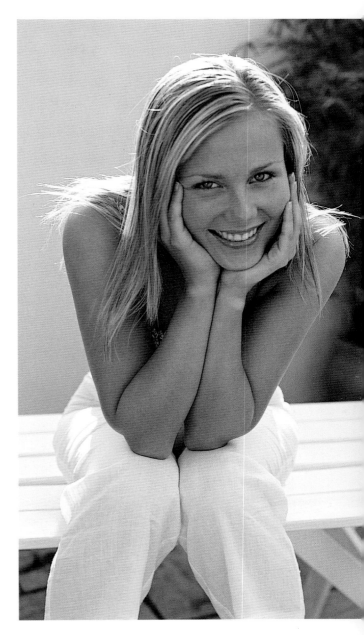

Tai chi is all about feeling good inside as well as outside.

the brim with our own egotistical thoughts and desires, all our prejudices and second-hand opinions, there will never be room for anything new or positive to enter our lives. Tai chi can help you let go of all that excess baggage, to make space inside for evolution and change to take place.

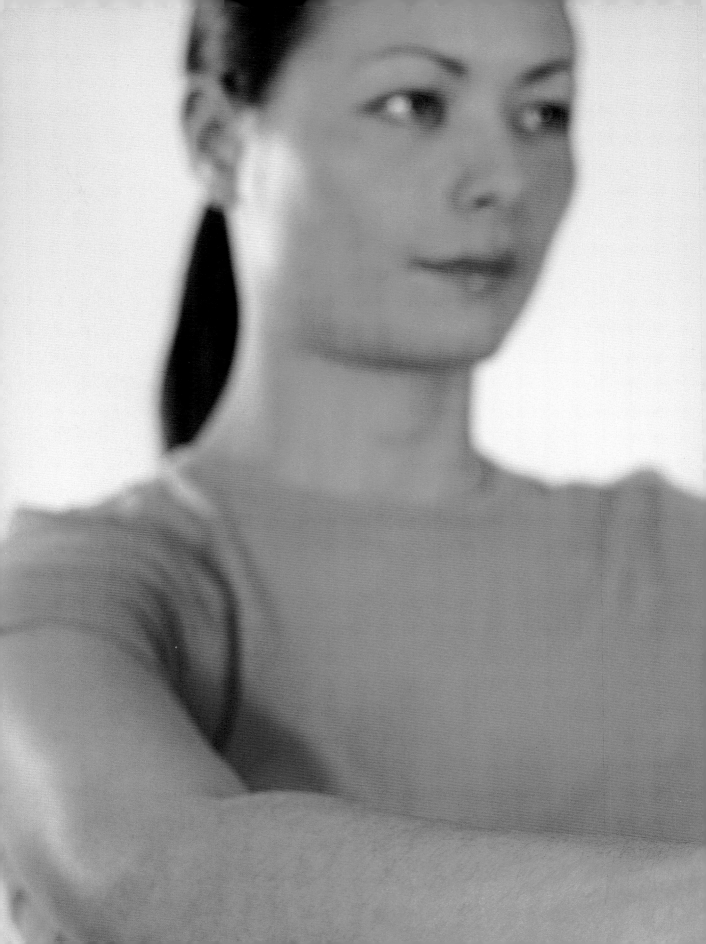

getting
started

When and Where to Practise

This chapter outlines a number of procedures and suggestions that will enable you
to progress more easily in your tai chi studies. The first of these focuses on the issue
of practice. Take a look at them before rushing off to do the movements themselves,
and refer back to them from time to time. They are important points and can make
the difference between success and failure.

The need to practise, and to practise regularly, are the
two most important things any teacher can impart to a
student. Without this commitment to practise, tai chi
cannot be learned, and anything that has been learned
will quickly be forgotten. This is as true for those just
starting out as it is for those who have been doing tai
chi for years. There are no short cuts to learning tai chi
and maintaining its wonderful benefits. Without regular
practice, all your efforts will be wasted.

WHEN TO PRACTISE
Traditionally, the best times to practise are early in the
morning or in the evening, when the energies of light
and dark (Yang and Yin) are considered to be in
harmony. For most people with a busy and often
irregular lifestyle, however, this is simply not possible.

You will need to find a daily rhythm that is right for
your own situation. Ideally, you should go through your
tai chi sequence at least once every day. As with most
commitments of this kind, sticking to a routine is best,
but ultimately, any time is better than never at all.

During the early months of study, you should aim to
learn one movement from this book each day, and make
a pledge to yourself that you will have it fully assimilated
before you finish your day and go to bed. In this way, you
add constantly to your repertoire of movements, until

> **REMEMBER!**
> Like most things that are worthwhile,
> tai chi takes time to master, and the main
> obstacles to success lie within yourself. By
> overcoming self-doubts, laziness and cynicism,
> you gain a very personal victory which is
> enduring and of immense value.

eventually, if you are patient and don't try to forge ahead
too quickly, you will become familiar with the whole
sequence. Then you can relax into the movements and
really begin to reap the rewards. It is worth the effort.

WHERE TO PRACTISE
This will be different for each person, depending on
your circumstances, but always look for the following
aspects in any practice space:

- **A clean, uncluttered space is essential.** You
  will need a minimum area of about 3 x 2 m (10 x 6 ft)
  in order to work right through the sequence from
  start to finish – more if you are quite tall.

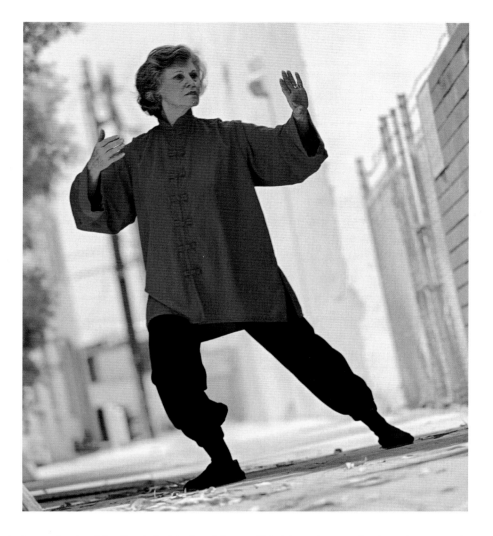

- **Fresh air is important – ideally, tai chi should be done outdoors.** Aim for this as soon as you feel confident with your movements. At the very least, ensure that your practice area is well ventilated. Traditionally, it is considered best to do tai chi in places where there is an abundance of natural energy – this usually means near to trees and/or running water – but any outdoor space is better than none. Certainly you should try to avoid obvious areas of pollution.

- **Always try to approach your sessions with a feeling of calm.** Make sure that your clothing is loose, comfortable and made from a natural fibre such as wool, cotton or silk. Ensure that your lower back and throat are kept warm and are protected from any adverse weather conditions such as wind or damp. Then aim to work for at least 10 minutes each time you practise.

Tai chi can be practised anytime, even in your lunch break.

- **Choose comfortable footwear, without too much of a heel.** If you are practising outdoors, your shoes need to be waterproof as well. Cold and damp can enter the body via the feet, and this can lead to illness, so keep them warm and dry. Make sure the fit is snug as this will enable you to balance more effectively than, say, loose sandals or slippers.

- **It is helpful if your practice sessions are undisturbed.** This is not always easy if you are sharing living space with others. However, do not be secretive about your tai chi studies, and if necessary explain to those around you what you are doing. Even if they are sceptical at first, they will become more supportive as they start to perceive the positive changes in you that tai chi can bring.

Posture and Stance

Let us now take a look at the various features of tai chi movement that make it so radically different to most other forms of exercise. These are associated to a large extent with the subject of posture and stance, of getting the body and limbs in just the right position and relationship, one to the other. It is important to understand this vital aspect of the work if you are to experience its lasting benefits.

Try to assimilate the details given in the remainder of this chapter now if you can, as it will make the learning process much easier. Also, if at any time you feel that things aren't going quite as well as you would like, or you are uncomfortable with any of the movements, refer back to these pages. You may find that you have misunderstood some aspect, or that there is something you are neglecting in your posture and stance.

KNEES

Whenever you watch somebody doing tai chi, you will notice that the centre of gravity is deliberately kept low, stealthy, almost cat-like in appearance. This is achieved by a deliberate and ample bend to the knees at all times. A degree of flexibility in the tendons of the hips, knees and inner thighs is cultivated, so that the stance can remain low-slung throughout the sequence – which typically will take around 8 minutes to complete.

This low stance greatly increases the aerobic quality of tai chi, and brings it into the realm of serious fitness training for those who wish to use it in this way. Even though the movements are still performed slowly, the low stance ensures a good workout. So never straighten your legs completely or lock the knees – the exception to this being if you are elderly or have stiff

legs. Here, it is perfectly acceptable to adapt the movements to a more erect, straightened posture. In time, your knees will become more flexible and you will be able to get down lower.

When you are standing in a forward stance , with most of your weight in the front leg, make sure that the

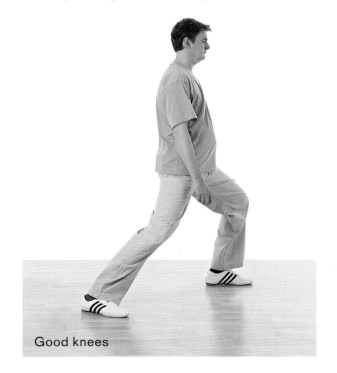

Good knees

knee does not extend beyond the tip of that foot. The photograph shows the right way to do this. If your knee drifts too far forward, you will immediately become off-balance. As a rule, if you look downwards to your front knee and beyond to the foot beneath it, you should just be able to see the very tips of your toes as your weight goes forward. Try not to go much further than that.

ELBOWS

Just as your knees should have a bend in them at all times, so too should your elbows. Never straighten your arms completely so that the elbows lock tightly: locked elbows mean muscular tension, and this will inhibit the flow of energy along your arms. Keep your elbows and wrists relaxed, with a little 'give' in them at all times. At the other extreme, try not to bend your elbows or wrists so much that sharp angles are created. This, too, will inhibit the flow of energy.

In other words, try to find a middle way where your arms, elbows, wrists and hands all present a pleasing, curvaceous appearance with a minimum of muscular tension.

SHOULDERS

It is essential to keep your shoulders relaxed as much as possible when doing tai chi – or, in fact, at any time.

Unfortunately, this is difficult for many people, but important to get right, because a tense neck and shoulders can inhibit the circulation of energy, blood and oxygen to your brain and interfere with your breathing.

So, let your shoulders drop. Lengthen your neck and breathe easily. Finally, try to maintain some free space under your armpits by keeping your arms and elbows away from your sides.

SPINE

Another main feature of posture that you will notice in tai chi is the straight back. The spinal column is held as erect as possible throughout the entire sequence. This is not achieved by adopting a stiff, punishing regime of tension and strain, or pulling in your shoulders and sucking in your tummy military style! It is achieved by doing just the opposite: the straight back is fashioned simply by relaxing your shoulders and drawing your bottom inwards. Your chin is then tucked in gently to lengthen your neck at the top, presenting a straight but relaxed appearance to the whole spinal column.

Think of the spine as a plumb line, hanging straight. In the classic texts on tai chi this is sometimes referred to as a 'golden thread suspended from heaven'. Imagine the spine being like this, so that whichever way you move, your body remains erect throughout.

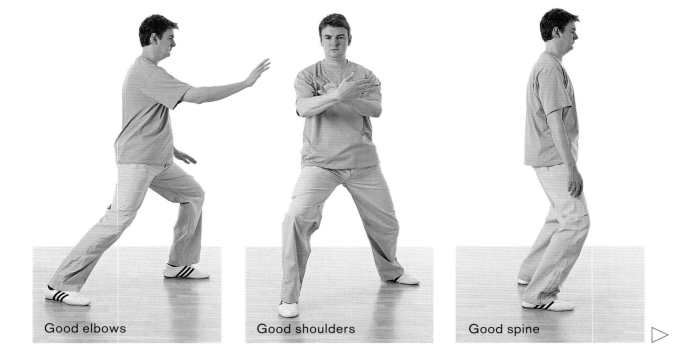

Good elbows

Good shoulders

Good spine

Keeping your root

Being 'rooted' is a concept that many people find curious, but it is central to tai chi practice. It relates, in part, to the existence of a major energy centre in the sole of the foot called the Bubbling Spring. This is a major acupuncture point with the ability to move energy downwards, suggesting that we can, indeed, discover and cultivate a way of being more intimately connected to the energies of the earth through the feet.

Bend your knees and sink down. Imagine roots extending down through your lower limbs and into the ground – great elastic roots that enable you to step from place to place, but which also keep you firmly balanced at all times. You may not feel any amazingly powerful sensation when you first try this, or even after a long period of practice. But it is there, and eventually most tai chi enthusiasts do come to understand what the concept of being rooted means, and how it feels. It will also assist you if you are engaged in dance or any sporting activity that requires balance and strength, from football to skiing.

Moving from the centre

When you first see tai chi being demonstrated, there appears to be a lot going on with the arms, but most often the apparently complex and large circular movements of the arms are achieved simply by turning the waist.

If you look closely at the photographs in this book, you will discover that the arms rarely stray far from a position just in front of the chest. Keep this in mind as you start to study the movements, and do not feel that you have to make large, extravagant gestures. Instead, try to keep space between your arms and your body, and then achieve as much as you can with your waist.

As you work, always strive to be aware of your centre – the Tan Tien (see page 14). Keep this area relaxed as you breathe in, even imagining the breath to be sinking down into your abdomen instead of going to your lungs (which are much higher up in the chest). The air will still go to your lungs, of course, but you will begin to establish an awareness of your vital centre lower down.

In addition, try to 'let go' and cultivate a sense of detachment from your conscious thoughts as you work – Wu Wei again (see page 23). All this can have enormous practical benefits over time and will really begin to make a difference to how you feel about your tai chi.

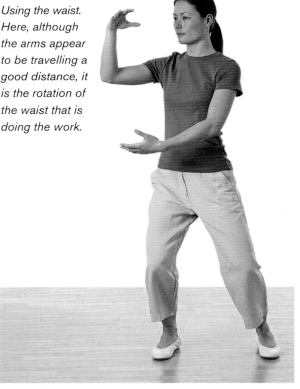

Using the waist. Here, although the arms appear to be travelling a good distance, it is the rotation of the waist that is doing the work.

Basic stances

Tai chi is all about continuous, uninterrupted movement – it is often described as being like a floating cloud or running stream. There are lots of steps between the movements, but there are also times when – even though your weight might be changing from side to side and your arms might be in motion all the time – your feet will remain fixed in one position.

There are usually just two ways in which the feet are placed at such times: wide stances and narrow stances. These terms will be used frequently in the instructions in this book, so you need to understand them clearly.

WIDE STANCES

Most of the stances in the tai chi sequence are termed 'wide stances' – or sometimes '70/30 stances', because that is usually the ratio of weight distribution: 70 per cent in the front foot, 30 per cent in the back, or vice versa.

A wide stance is one in which the feet are placed 'shoulder-width' apart – that is, the distance from one shoulder tip to the other. Do not confuse this with length, which can vary. You will have one foot ahead of the other, creating the length of the stance, but it is the width between the feet that is important.

Typical wide stances occur in movements such as Ward Off (see page 46) and Separate Hands and Push (see page 50).

NARROW STANCES

There are many stances in which most of your weight resides in one side or is concentrated in just one leg. The weighted side or 'substantial leg' is always the back leg, or foot. The front foot, meanwhile, rests lightly upon the ground, making light contact with either the heel or the toes. Typically, about 10 per cent of your weight will be residing in that front foot, with the rest in the back, substantial leg. When this occurs, the stance becomes narrower than in wide stances, and your front foot is placed ahead of and roughly in line with your back heel. The back foot is also usually turned out at a generous and comfortable angle to lend a firm base of support.

Typical narrow stances occur in movements such as Crane Spreads its Wings (see page 56) and Play Guitar (see page 54).

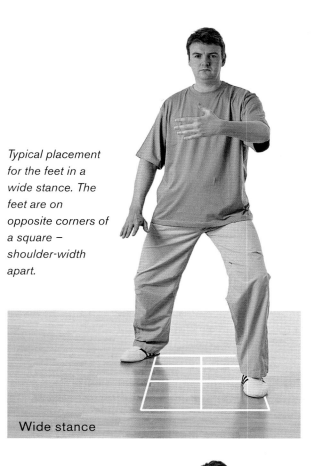

Typical placement for the feet in a wide stance. The feet are on opposite corners of a square – shoulder-width apart.

Wide stance

Typical placement for the feet in a narrow stance. The feet are on the corners of the rectangle as before – but you can see that the rectangle is much narrower than the previous one.

Narrow stance

Changing Positions and Stepping

Tai chi is all about movement, of getting around from one position to the next – and doing this as slowly and as gracefully as possible. We do not fall or stumble into any of the movements, but endeavour to glide smoothly, and to place the feet firmly all the way through from start to finish. It is useful, therefore, to know how to change position and step from one movement into the next with the minimum of effort.

Before you take any step, make sure your weight is settled in the substantial leg. This is the one that will remain stationary and bear your weight. Then lift the other foot – sometimes called the 'empty foot' – slowly off the ground; test your balance for a second and then step out. Remember that in tai chi you will be moving far more slowly than you are used to and therefore your balance is crucial to managing the steps smoothly.

After each step into a wide stance, it is usually advisable to adjust the back foot to a new, more comfortable position. For instance, if you have stepped around 90 degrees with the right foot, then the left foot (which has borne your weight) will still be pointing out in its original direction, possibly at an uncomfortable angle, so you need to adjust it at the end of the manoeuvre by pivoting inwards on the heel. A good example occurs early in the sequence for Grasp the Bird's Tail (see page 47), where at the end of the movement the back foot pivots into a comfortable position as the weight goes forward.

When stepping into a narrow stance, you will need to adjust what is to become the back foot before you step. This foot will be bearing most of your weight at the end of the placement and obviously

you cannot move it *then*. A good example of this can be seen on page 56, where the right foot has been adjusted inwards by pivoting on the heel, before the narrow heel stance of Crane Spreads its Wings is created. The weight can then settle comfortably in the right foot while the left toes make the narrow stance.

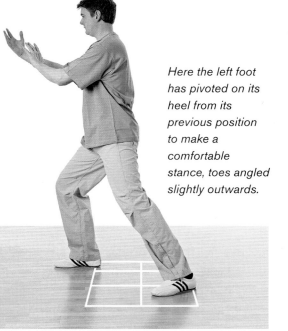

Here the left foot has pivoted on its heel from its previous position to make a comfortable stance, toes angled slightly outwards.

Hand Shapes and Movements

During the tai chi sequence, there are certain hand shapes that crop up again and again, each one shaping and directing the internal energy in its own unique way. There are numerous subtle variations on these, producing the rich variety of movement that makes up the tai chi experience, but these are not as complicated as they might first appear. It is well worth looking at the most basic shapes now.

HOLDING THE BALL

This shape makes use of both hands, as if embracing a ball or balloon. The size of the ball can vary, but usually the hands are positioned opposite each other – for instance, with the left hand on top while the right hand supports the ball from beneath. The hands themselves also present a curved aspect, as though resting on a spherical surface. See also pages 45 and 88.

PUSH

The hand in this position makes a shape as if pushing outwards. Sometimes both hands make the push together, but usually it is just one. See also pages 57 and 131.

FLAT HAND

In this position, the hand is held in a rather flat aspect, the fingers pointing upwards. Be careful not to create any tension as you do this. Keep your fingers relaxed, never locked tight. See also pages 48 and 79.

BRUSHING HAND

This occurs in certain stepping movements, where the hand is called upon figuratively to 'brush' across the knee or thigh from the centre outwards. The palm faces downwards during this movement and stays at

Holding the ball

Push

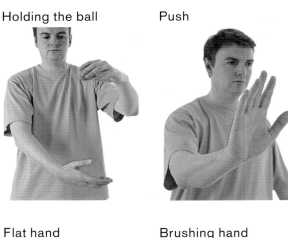

Flat hand

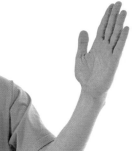

Brushing hand

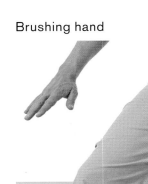

a good distance from the knee as it passes. Keep the wrist relaxed as you do this, but never floppy or limp. See also pages 59 and 104.

Warm-ups

In a sense, any warm-up exercise that gently frees the joints and tendons is suitable, but those illustrated here are particularly useful for tai chi. They are mostly repetitive movements, so are quite different in character to the tai chi form itself. However, what they do have in common is the aim of opening up and clearing stagnation and tension from the joints and tendons, thereby allowing the energy to flow more smoothly.

You should aim to spend at least 2–3 minutes on warm-ups before commencing the tai chi form. This way, you will gain the maximum benefit from the form itself. If you are doing tai chi outdoors in cool weather, these warm-ups become especially important and you can stay with them for a little longer if you like.

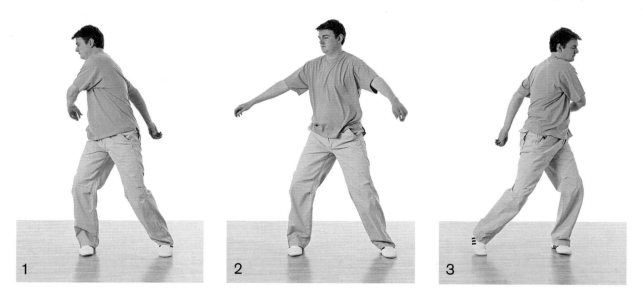

1

2

3

TWISTING

With your feet wide apart, a good bend to your knees and your arms hanging loose, rotate your waist first one way then the other, alternating from side to side. Allow your arms to flop around, very relaxed and empty like a 'rag doll', so that they tend to wind themselves around your waist as you go. Keep your knees apart at all times and do not allow them to 'cave in' towards each other with the turning of your body. Also keep plenty of space under your armpits. Build up a rhythm.

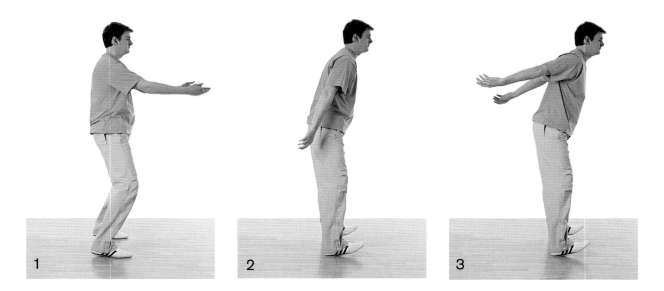

ROCKING

With your knees bent and shoulders relaxed, rock gently back and forth on your feet by raising your heels and then your toes alternately (like somebody wearing banana-shaped shoes). As you do this, allow your arms to pitch back and forth as well: forward and up, then behind. Your arms swing forward as your heels lift, and then back behind as your toes lift. Do not feel discouraged if it takes a while to get used to this kind of movement. Again, try to get a good, steady rhythm going, and remember to bend those knees! This way, you will stay balanced.

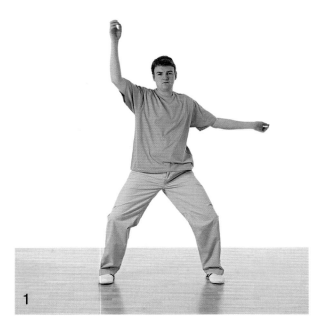

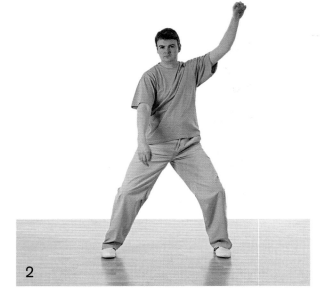

SHOULDER ROLLS

Making sure you have lots of space above and to the sides, circle your arms up and around several times, loosening your shoulders. As you roll your arms, alternate them as if swimming; do this slowly, with your elbows relaxed and loose. Then change the direction of the roll, still alternating in a swimming motion but this time as if doing a backstroke. Finally, shake your arms vigorously, trying to get that shaking sensation to extend right up from your hands to your shoulders. Make sure you have enough space to do this without hitting your hands on anything.

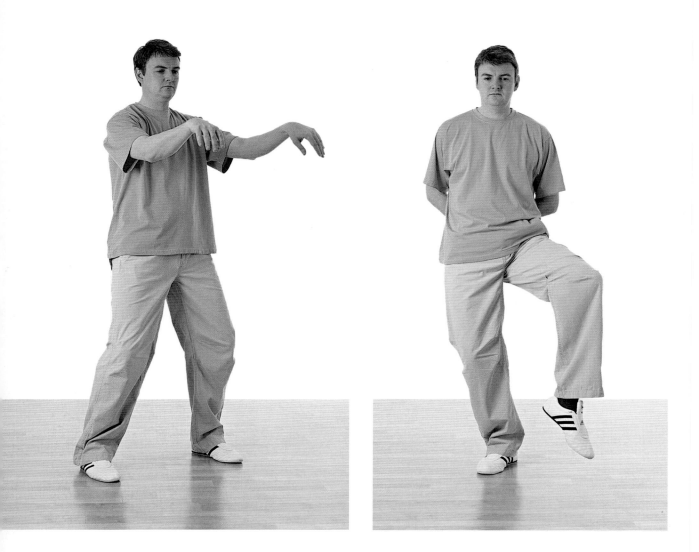

WRIST ROTATIONS

Extend your arms in front of you and allow your wrists to drop, so that your fingers are pointing downwards. Then rotate your hands slowly, as if stirring, around and around, gently and without tension. Do this a minimum of 10 times in one direction, then reverse and do roughly the same number of rotations the other way. Finally, shake out your hands vigorously (as if you had a sticky toffee paper clinging to each finger). Shake and loosen your hands. Repeat the exercise if necessary and shake again.

FOOT ROTATIONS

This is similar to the previous exercise, but this time you rotate your feet. Raise one knee to lift the foot from the ground, then slowly rotate the ankle. The toes remain pointing downwards throughout. Do this a minimum of 10 times in one direction, then reverse and do roughly the same number of rotations the other way. Initially, if your balance is poor you can support yourself against a chair or wall. Finally, shake the whole foot vigorously to shift any congestion or tension in the ankle joint. Place the foot down slowly, raise your other knee and repeat with the other foot, rotating both ways and then shaking out as before.

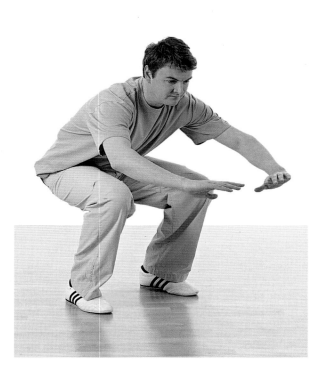

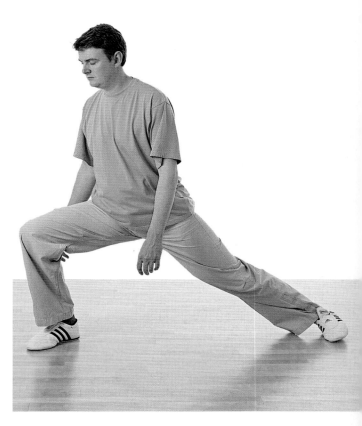

SQUAT

For this, simply squat down on both feet with your knees close together. Do not go down too far at first; instead, build up the depth of your squat by degrees. Use a chair for support if necessary. This is an excellent exercise for loosening your knees. Once your flexibility and balance improve, try it with your heels flat on the ground, too. Repeat several times, then shake out your legs one at a time with a little kicking and shaking motion, to clear any tension.

LEG STRETCHES

Go easy on these, especially if you are not particularly flexible, and make sure you do not support your weight by leaning on your own thigh at any stage. Separate your feet as wide as is comfortable and then sink down, first on one side and then the other, to stretch the inner aspect of each leg alternately. Experiment with different ways of doing this, to stretch different parts of the leg. Rather than forcing yourself to stretch too far, simply do lots of gentle repetitions of the stretch, to loosen everything up gradually and without strain.

How to Use This Book

The Short Yang Form of tai chi as created and passed down by Master Chen Man Ch'ing in the middle part of the last century is normally taught in two sections, called parts 1 and 2. Each of these parts has its own distinct beginning and end. You can see this division clearly in this book because we are using different models – a man for part 1 and a woman for part 2.

Part 1 is what most beginners aim for, and will provide around 2 minutes of movement. **Part 2** is more challenging and adds a further 6 minutes. Within the form there is also a short sequence, repeated several times, that we refer to here as the Chorus, and there are also definite changes in the character of the movements as you progress through the form.

Do not worry if you find you are working through the whole form in less than 8 minutes. The most important thing is that you keep to your own natural pace of breathing, and enjoy it.

You are now almost ready to begin learning the tai chi sequence. When using the instructions for the movements in the rest of this book, you will need to bear in mind the points on the opposite page.

MOVEMENT TYPES

Early movements of the form are all about developing balance and becoming aware of your own personal space.

Narrow stances help to develop balance and are excellent preparation for the 'kicks' that follow later.

Diagonal steps encourage you to orient yourself much more in relation to your own centre.

Stepping backwards and sideways challenges you to use the space behind you, an area which you cannot see and which we are usually completely unaware of. It also features some interesting lateral movements.

Downwards and upwards movements dip down and rise up again and include 'kicks', encouraging you to focus on staying 'rooted'.

Rotational movements call upon your ability to rotate and turn, moving through diagonals or circles. Here you are really starting to 'fly' and enjoy your tai chi to the full.

The Chorus is a series of movements that occurs four times through the form and helps greatly with the task of memorizing the whole routine.

The closing steps bring the whole sequence to an end with a flamboyant flourish that integrates and progresses those skills already learned.

USING THE FLOOR GRID

You will notice that a floor grid of white squares has been superimposed on some of the photographs in the instruction pages that follow. This is particularly helpful for indicating the orientation of the feet, one to the other. For example, sometimes a movement calls for the front foot to be pointing directly ahead, while the rear foot is turned out at an angle, and this can be seen clearly by referring to the grid.

The white squares are also helpful for establishing that all-important distance between your feet, and especially the width between them during wide stances. Consider the squares to be roughly 20 x 20 cm (8 x 8 in) each. This means that two squares together are roughly 'shoulder width', and so equal to the distance between your feet in any typical wide stance, depending on your size and height. If you are tall, you can think of the squares as being proportionally larger.

Note that the grid cannot show the distances between one step and the other over several movements – it would have to be very large indeed to achieve that. As we have seen, the overall area needed for the whole form is 3 x 2 m (10 x 6 ft), and a floor grid of that size would take up a whole page if it were shown in full. So don't be tempted to compare them!

When you reach your third repetition of the Chorus (see page 107), after a lengthy sequence of stepping forward into wide stances all in the same direction, you might, if working indoors, begin to run out of space. Try stepping wide rather than significantly forward to save space. Later, when you have learned the sequence and you venture outdoors, you can return to long steps as shown in the photographs.

WEIGHT DISTRIBUTION

Alongside the photographs you will find indications for the distribution of weight. Just one foot is indicated in each photo, but 70 per cent in the right foot means, by definition, that there will be 30 per cent in the left. Don't become too fixated on this: these percentages are just guidelines. The main thing is that you feel relaxed and properly balanced at all times. Make sure you have the correct width between your feet and the rest will usually fall into place naturally.

BREATHING

Guidelines are also provided as to how the movements co-ordinate with the breath. Remember that the tai chi form is shaped around your natural rhythm of breathing, and that rhythm remains even and regular throughout. Never force your breath into any pattern that feels uncomfortable for you. Just use your own pattern and your own rhythm, no matter how fast or slow it seems to begin with, then simply aim to fit the movements around that natural rhythm.

As you will discover once you start using the instructions and photographs, there is almost always one whole cycle of breath (in and out) for each movement. Two photographs are usually sufficient to depict each cycle: one to cover the in-breath aspect, the other the out-breath. However, in some instances where the movement is particularly intricate, more photographs may have been used. Where this occurs, remember that the rhythm remains constant. In other words, the inhalation does not take longer just because there might, for example, be two photographs to show it instead of one. Think of a piece of music, with a regular rhythm that does not alter. That is your tai chi form, with the rhythm being your breath. Shape the movements around that rhythm, and stay comfortable at all times.

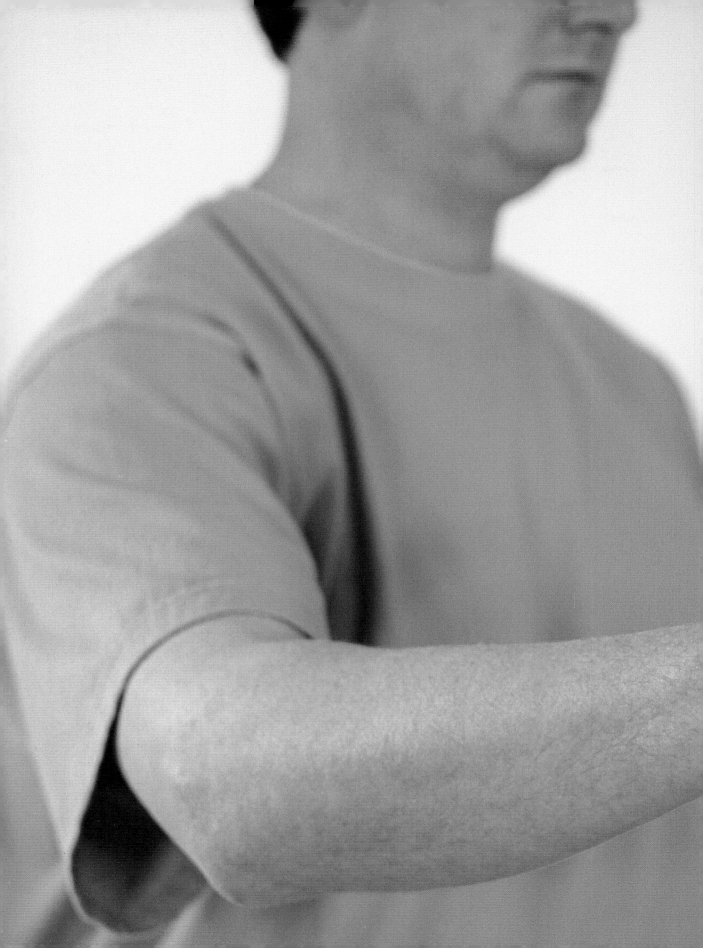

the
short yang
form

Part 1

Preparation

Beginnings are important. You need to feel comfortable and also calm. Sink down a little and allow your knees to bend. Relax your shoulders. This is a special moment, full of possibilities, before the Yang and the Yin divide and are set in motion. Wait for the right time to begin.

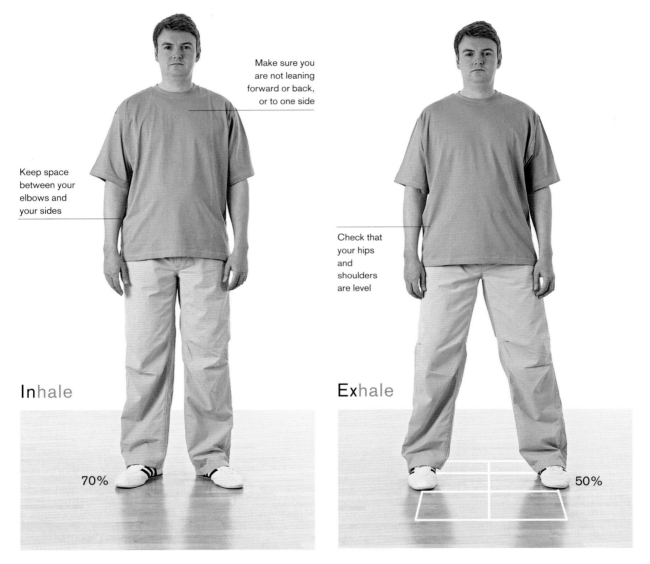

Make sure you are not leaning forward or back, or to one side

Keep space between your elbows and your sides

Check that your hips and shoulders are level

Inhale

70%

Exhale

50%

BEGIN BY standing upright with your feet together, the heels not quite touching.

1 Sink most of your weight into your right foot by slowly emptying the weight from your left side. Then begin to raise your left foot from the ground.

2 Slide your left foot further to the left, to set it down shoulder width from your right with the toes pointing forwards. Then adjust the toes of your right foot so that they also point forwards. Your weight then settles evenly into both feet. Notice that your feet are actually parallel to each other at this stage.

Opening

The Opening of the form has your weight evenly placed in both feet and provides an excellent opportunity to establish a good, regular rhythm to your breathing. Some people like to repeat it several times until they feel calm and centred within. Try to let your arms 'float' slowly through the movements, without tension.

BEGIN BY relaxing and trying to let go of any tension or negativity inside. Take as long as you like.

 With your wrists relaxed and loose, allow your arms to 'float' upwards to about chest height, your forearms parallel with the ground, wrists relaxed and fingers pointing slightly downwards.

Make sure your palms do not appear to lift and push forward

Do not straighten your fingers completely

Keep your shoulders low and relaxed as you raise your arms

Exhale

Inhale

50%

50%

2 Gradually 'drop' your wrists so that your fingers appear to straighten and point forwards – this is preferable to raising your fingers physically. See how slowly you can do this without your fingers trembling or tensing up.

Avoid tension in your upper back, between your shoulder blades

3 Still keeping space between your elbows and your sides, slowly draw back your elbows. Keep your shoulders relaxed as you do this, and maintain an upright spine throughout. Do not lean backwards. Remember, only your arms should move.

Inhale

50%

Keep your wrists relaxed and soft

Exhale

50%

4 Slowly place your hands back down to your sides and let your knees bend just a little as you sink down and breathe out. It sometimes helps to imagine pushing a ball down through water as you do this (but without using any muscular tension), giving your hands a soft, rounded appearance.

Turn Right

Here we first meet with the idea of 'holding a ball' – a certain presence between the hands. Even though you will discover that the size of the ball varies from place to place, this subtle energy connection between the palms is rarely absent throughout the entire form. Here the ball is quite large.

BEGIN BY emptying the weight from your right side and sinking into your left foot.

1 Raise the toes of your right foot and then pivot on the heel to turn the foot clockwise to the right. At the same time, begin to raise your right arm while simultaneously drawing up your left palm just a little, as if supporting a large ball from beneath. The right palm, meanwhile, rests on top of the ball.

2 Place all of your right foot flat on to the ground and slowly bring your weight into it. If you look down, your knee will appear to go just over the tip of your toes as you bend it. Otherwise, your gaze should be directed outwards, looking just over your right hand, as if towards a distant horizon.

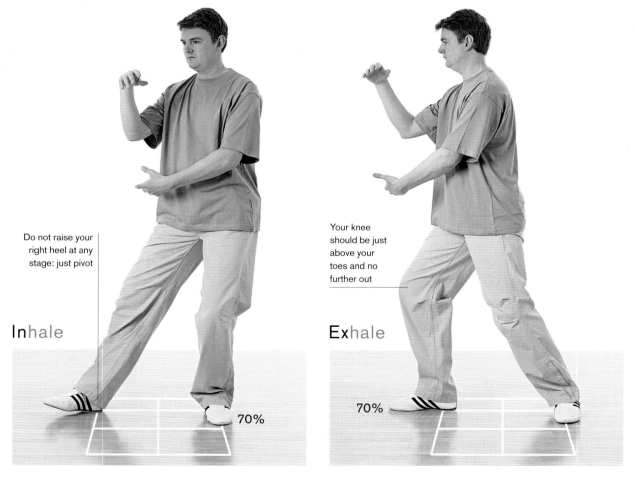

Do not raise your right heel at any stage: just pivot

Your knee should be just above your toes and no further out

Inhale

Exhale

70%

70%

Ward Off

Here we meet with the first wide 70/30 stance of the sequence. Wide stances feature strongly over the next few pages, as you keep your feet shoulder-width apart when stepping, regardless of any length between one foot and the other.

BEGIN BY transferring your weight into your right side while drawing in the toes of your left foot slightly towards your right heel.

1 With your left foot raised slightly, check your balance and prepare to step out by sinking down into the back foot. During the Ward Off, your hands do what is called 'palming'. This is where the surfaces of the palms figuratively 'stroke' each other at a distance, the one rising as the other falls. Get ready for this by uncurling your right hand slightly to show your palm, ready to 'stroke' downwards.

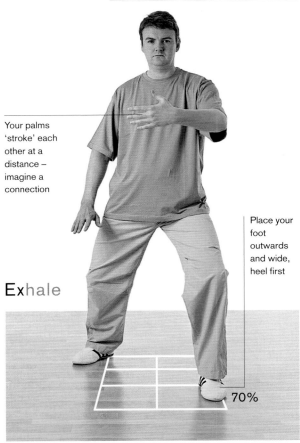

Your palms 'stroke' each other at a distance – imagine a connection

Place your foot outwards and wide, heel first

Exhale

70%

Sink down into your right heel for balance

Inhale

100%

2 Step out with your left foot and bend your left knee as your weight goes forward. At the same time, your left forearm should rise to a horizontal position in front of your chest, palm in, while your right hand falls to your side, palm back. Your centre now faces forwards again, as at the start. Finally, adjust what is now your back foot by pivoting a little on your right heel, to release any tension in the knee.

Grasp the Bird's Tail

If you ever watch an expert holding a racing pigeon, you will recognize the shape of the hands here. This movement marks the beginning of your first Chorus (see pages 38–39), which continues through to the Single Whip on pages 51–53. The sequence is repeated several times in the tai chi form, like a chorus in a piece of music.

(see pages 38–39)

BENEFITS

• The generous movements of your waist help to tone your waistline.

• This also stimulates the energy centres clustered in that area and from which all movements, in any physical activity, can be directed more effectively.

BEGIN BY shifting your weight to the left and drawing the toes of your right foot inwards a little towards your left heel.

1 Turn your waist slightly to your left and pick up an imaginary ball, with your left hand on top and your right hand supporting from underneath. Do not take the image of the 'ball' too literally – it is used just to get you started. In time, when all the movements begin to feel natural, you can discard the image of the ball and think simply of energy.

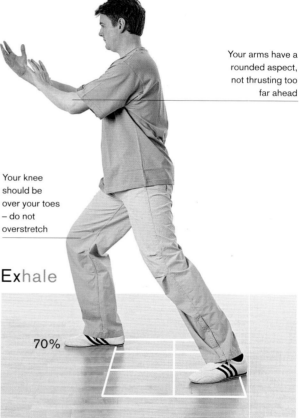

Your arms have a rounded aspect, not thrusting too far ahead

Your knee should be over your toes – do not overstretch

Exhale

70%

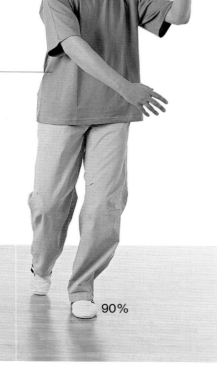

Your waist moves slightly counter-clockwise

Inhale

90%

2 Rotating your waist clockwise this time, step around to your right, heel first, into a wide stance. Bend your right knee to bring your weight forward and adjust your back foot to a comfortable position by pivoting on your left heel. The 'ball' goes with you but it becomes smaller, so that your right arm finishes in a position slanting upwards and to the right, while the fingers of your left hand point slightly upwards towards your right palm, at about chest height.

Rollback and Press

These two movements are treated together here, since they share one breath and therefore one complete round of Yin and Yang. Again, your waist plays an important part in shaping the movements, rotating first a little clockwise, then counter-clockwise, before turning back to face forwards again with another clockwise rotation.

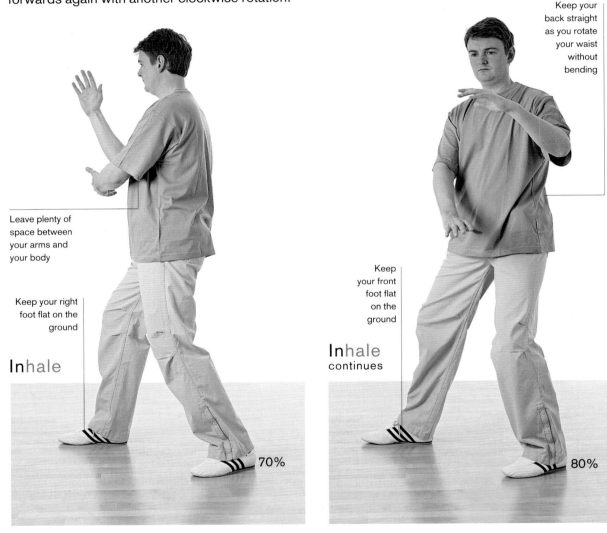

Leave plenty of space between your arms and your body

Keep your right foot flat on the ground

Inhale

70%

Keep your back straight as you rotate your waist without bending

Keep your front foot flat on the ground

Inhale
continues

80%

BEGIN BY shifting most of your weight into your back leg.

1 Rotate or 'roll' your hands slightly while sliding your left palm, at a distance, down your right forearm to a position just beside your elbow. Meanwhile, the angle of your right elbow has become more acute, so that your forearm is almost pointing upwards. During all this, rotate your waist slightly clockwise, with your arms following slightly to the right as well.

2 Still with your inhalation, rotate your waist counter-clockwise and draw your left hand back and around, left of centre, while your right forearm folds down almost horizontal. Most of your weight is now in your back leg. Try to cultivate a feeling of contact between your hands even though they remain separated. Keep thinking of that energetic connection from one arm to the other as you go.

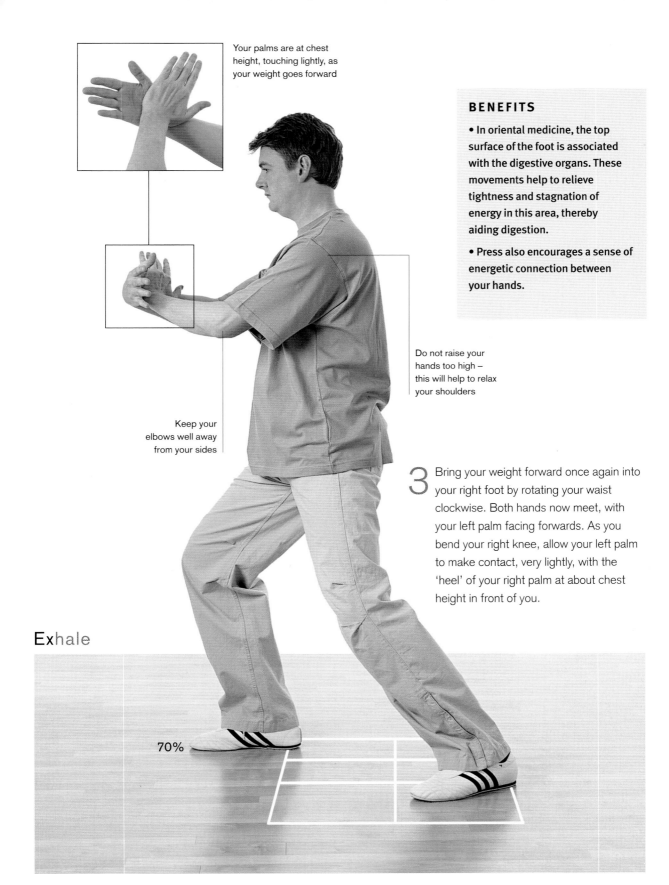

Your palms are at chest height, touching lightly, as your weight goes forward

BENEFITS

• In oriental medicine, the top surface of the foot is associated with the digestive organs. These movements help to relieve tightness and stagnation of energy in this area, thereby aiding digestion.

• Press also encourages a sense of energetic connection between your hands.

Do not raise your hands too high – this will help to relax your shoulders

Keep your elbows well away from your sides

3 Bring your weight forward once again into your right foot by rotating your waist clockwise. Both hands now meet, with your left palm facing forwards. As you bend your right knee, allow your left palm to make contact, very lightly, with the 'heel' of your right palm at about chest height in front of you.

Exhale

70%

Separate Hands and Push

The name of this movement is very descriptive of what takes place, but it should be done without leaning your body forwards or backwards at any stage. Although leaning into a movement is encouraged in some styles of tai chi, in the Short Yang Form you try to keep an upright spine throughout.

BEGIN BY letting go of the previous formation of your hands and rolling your palms into a downward-facing position.

BENEFITS

• This sequence is excellent for stimulating Lung energy. The thumbs play an important part: in oriental medicine, the energy of the Lungs surfaces in the chest and finishes in the thumbs.

1 Separate your hands horizontally with a little 'swimming' motion, outwards and back, with your thumbs pointing towards your chest. As you separate your hands, imagine a connection between the breathing process and your thumbs. At the same time, transfer your weight into your rear foot. Don't lean back as you do this. If you suspect that this is happening, sink downwards instead.

2 Rotate your hands so that the palms are facing outwards, then bring your weight forward by bending your right knee. The appearance of the 'push' comes from your hands and is made by bending your knees, not thrusting forward with your arms. Remember not to lean into the push: keep in mind the internal plumb line (see page 29), and keep your back straight. As you exhale, let go mentally of any tension in your chest.

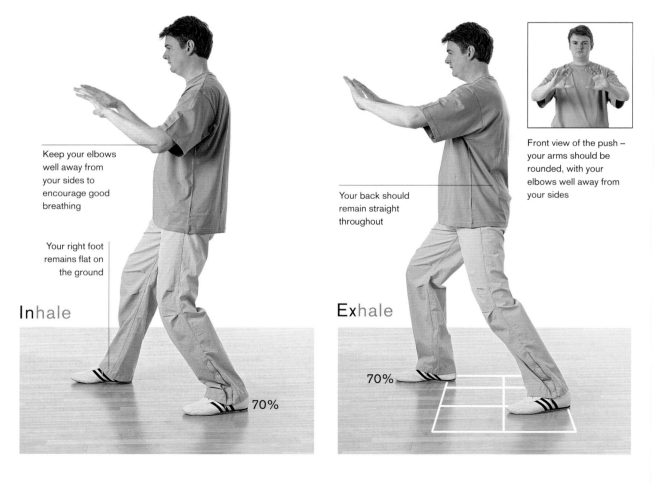

Keep your elbows well away from your sides to encourage good breathing

Your right foot remains flat on the ground

Inhale

70%

Your back should remain straight throughout

Exhale

70%

Front view of the push – your arms should be rounded, with your elbows well away from your sides

Single Whip

This is an important movement that is repeated several times in the tai chi form. The term 'whip' comes from a rippling, whip-like movement of the arm that is apparent in the traditional Long Form of tai chi. Although this is no longer obvious here in the Short Form, the name has stuck.

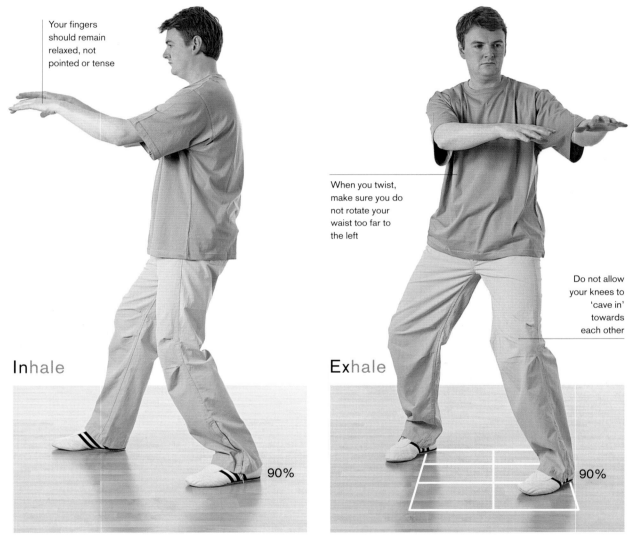

Your fingers should remain relaxed, not pointed or tense

When you twist, make sure you do not rotate your waist too far to the left

Do not allow your knees to 'cave in' towards each other

Inhale

90%

Exhale

90%

BEGIN BY shifting most of your weight into your back leg and allowing your arms to relax.

1 Your hands flatten with palms down, and you should find that your arms extend naturally without effort as you straighten your right knee. Just sit back and relax into the movement. Keep your elbows soft, with a little 'give' in your arms at all times.

2 Keeping your arms in the same outstretched position, slowly rotate your centre counter-clockwise by pivoting on your right heel. Your feet should become slightly 'pigeon-toed' – as if placed on the sides of a triangle. At the end of this turn, both feet should be flat on the ground, but with your weight now mostly in your left side.

The Crane's Beak:
allow your wrist to relax,
thumb and index finger in
very light contact.

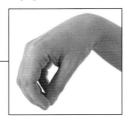

3 Draw your right hand inwards closer to your body,
allowing your right elbow to bend and go 'sharper'.
Next, rotate your waist clockwise and allow your
weight to drift back into your right side. Meanwhile,
your right hand forms itself into a 'crane's beak', a
distinctive bunching-up of the fingers and thumb.
Think of taking up a pinch of sand – just light enough
for fingers and thumb to be in contact but not tense.

Your eyes follow
the crane's beak
but your head
stays centred

Inhale

90%

The weight remains
predominantly in your
right foot, allowing the
toes of your left foot
to pivot freely

Exhale

90%

4 If the previous movement felt like gently
coiling a spring, then this is where we let
the spring go! Project your crane's beak
outwards, just right of centre, until your
arm is almost straight. At the same time,
pivot on the toes of your left foot and rotate
your centre counter-clockwise. Try to keep
your chin in line with your breastbone and
navel – everything centred.

5 Sink all your weight into your right foot, preparing to step way around to your far left. This is a big step, so make sure your balance is established before you raise your left foot from the ground. You may find it helpful to draw the toes of your left foot inwards a little towards your right heel before you finally step out. By this time, your left hand should be rising from a position close to your right hip.

Check your balance now, before the big step

In hale

100%

BENEFITS

• **This is an excellent toning exercise for your waist, and a test of flexibility and balance.**

• **It encourages relaxation in your wrists and elbows, and gently stimulates the tendons and ligaments of the knees and ankles.**

• **The gentle stimulation and opening of the lower right side helps to prevent a build-up of stagnant Liver chi, which is implicated in health problems from migraine headaches to premenstrual syndrome.**

Adjust what has now become the back foot by pivoting on your right heel

Your left knee should be over your left toes at the finish

Ex hale

70%

6 Step around to your far left, making contact with your left heel first and then bending your left knee as your weight settles forward. Your left hand rises and rotates as you go, to finish with the palm and fingers facing straight ahead, in front of your left breast, with your elbow relaxed. Meanwhile, your right arm remains extended and slightly behind you, the crane's beak still intact. Adjust your back foot at the end of the movement to make sure you are comfortable.

Play Guitar

The tai chi sequence continues with a movement in which you meet with a narrow stance for the first time. As outlined on page 31, with narrow stances most of the weight goes into your back leg, with your front foot positioned just lightly in contact with the ground. These stances are excellent for developing balance.

BENEFITS

• This narrow stance improves your balance, helping you to maintain a sense of internal equilibrium and better concentration.

• The movement helps to unite the energies of two important acu-points, in the palm and the wrist, which are particularly calming in nature.

BEGIN BY Letting go of the crane's beak in your right hand. Then make a small adjustment of your left foot by pivoting inwards on your left heel – not too far, but just sufficient to take the pressure off what is to become your back leg.

1 Raise your right heel by pivoting on your toes. Open your arms a little, like a bird about to flap its wings, while simultaneously transferring all your weight into your left foot and rotating your waist clockwise. You are in the process of turning 90 degrees to your right.

Try to feel an energetic connection between your arms as they approach each other

Your elbows should be lower than your wrists

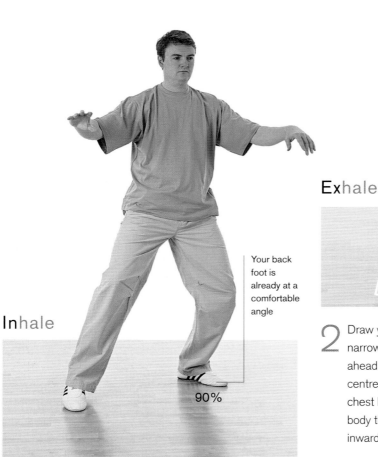

Inhale

Your back foot is already at a comfortable angle

90%

Exhale

90%

2 Draw your right heel across to place it down in a narrow heel stance, hips and shoulders facing straight ahead. Meanwhile, your arms drift closer to your centre, your right arm extended outwards at about chest height while your left palm, a little nearer to your body than the right, settles in a position 'looking' inwards towards your right forearm.

Pull and Step with Shoulder

This movement is rare in tai chi because it finishes with the body facing away from the direction of the leading foot. Usually, your centre (navel), hips and shoulders, and chin will all be nicely squared up and facing in the direction of your front foot. Here, however, there is a subtle twist at the end of the movement.

BEGIN BY letting go of the Play Guitar shape in your arms and placing all your weight into your back foot.

1 Lower your arms together in a pulling motion. The left hand drifts a little behind at about waist height, left of centre, while your right arm drops almost vertically across the middle of your body, fingers pointing downwards. As you do this, rotate your waist slightly counter-clockwise and draw in the toes of your right foot, to place them just ahead of your left heel.

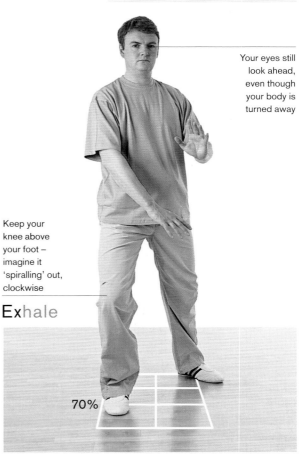

Your eyes still look ahead, even though your body is turned away

Keep your knee above your foot – imagine it 'spiralling' out, clockwise

Exhale

70%

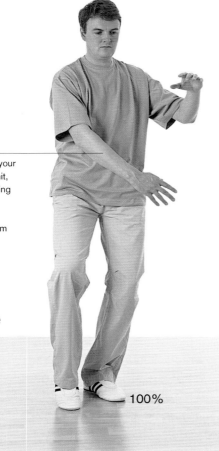

Try to move your arms as a unit, still maintaining the energy connection between them

Inhale

100%

2 Step forward into a wide stance with your right foot, heel first, and bend your knee. Throughout, maintain the counter-clockwise turn in your waist, so that your right shoulder appears to project forward. Your right arm stays roughly where it was a moment ago, while your left hand settles at about waist height, palm facing forwards slightly and still maintaining a subtle energy connection with your right forearm.

Crane Spreads its Wings

The crane has a special significance in oriental culture and philosophy, representing strength and gracefulness. Together, these make for a very special combination, something to which the tai chi student should always aspire. Here, with this elegant movement, it is the right foot that supports your weight.

BENEFITS

• Said to stimulate the central nervous system through the upright aspect of the spine.

• It also closely resembles certain chi kung postures that stimulate the digestive energies.

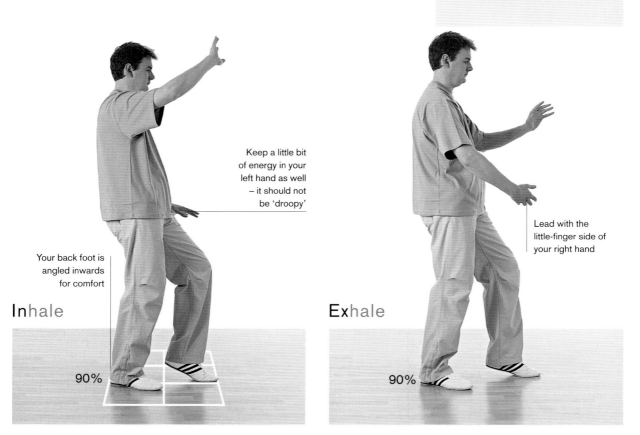

Keep a little bit of energy in your left hand as well – it should not be 'droopy'

Your back foot is angled inwards for comfort

Inhale

90%

Lead with the little-finger side of your right hand

Exhale

90%

BEGIN BY adjusting what is to become the back, weighted foot by pivoting inwards a little on your right heel.

1 With your weight in your right foot, rotate your centre counter-clockwise and form a narrow toe stance with your left foot, which will be aligned towards your right heel. Meanwhile, your left hand drops, to hover above your left thigh, while your right hand rises to about head height, palm outwards and upward-facing, so that your arms become like great wings. Your right hand also looks like somebody shielding their eyes from the sun.

2 Next, and while keeping your feet in the same position, change the wings! Lower your right arm to about hip height, while simultaneously lifting your left hand so that it rises and sweeps around in front of your centre. Your arms should move in graceful curves – rather like turning a giant wheel – so that you can maintain that subtle energy connection between the palms as they go. Focus your energies in your right arm and particularly the little-finger side of your right arm, as you lead it slowly downwards.

Brush Knee and Push

Like so many descriptions used in tai chi, the name of this movement is not to be taken too literally. You do not brush the knee, but rather drift across it with your palm at a distance. The whole thing is a natural continuation of the wide circular movements of the crane's wings, with lots of space between your arms and body.

BEGIN BY rotating your waist clockwise.

1 Allow that right 'wing' to circle back, right of centre, palm up. At the same time, your left hand continues to circle up, over and down across your centre. If you were to trace the course of your left hand through the previous movement and into this, it would appear to be making a vertical, clockwise circle in front of you.

Allow your eyes to focus softly on your right palm as it drifts back

Keep your shoulders properly aligned with your hips

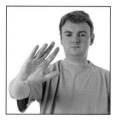

Your right palm is almost central, roughly in line with your right breast, not drifting too far out to the side

Keep your hand about 20 cm (8 in) from your knee throughout the movement

Exhale

70%

Inhale

100%

2 Take a step sideways and slightly forwards with your left foot, away from your narrow stance and into a wide one. Your left knee goes over the toes of your left foot as your weight shifts forward. As you step, 'brush' across your left knee with your left palm from right to left. Finally, push forward with your right palm at about chest height.

Play Guitar, left

Next, we are going to repeat a movement already learned – Play Guitar (see page 54). This movement is the same, but performed on the other side, with the left foot leading. The hands are reversed as well. Here, too, we get our first glimpse of the tai chi technique of stepping backwards.

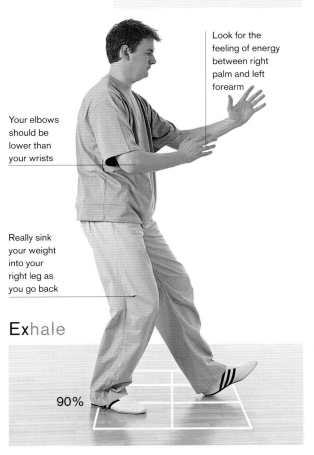

BENEFITS

• This narrow stance improves your balance, helping you to maintain a sense of internal equilibrium and better concentration.

• The movement helps to unite the energies of two important acu-points, in the palm and the wrist.

BEGIN BY bringing all your weight into your left foot, allowing the back foot to leave the ground.

1 Relax your hands and bring your right foot forward off the ground – this looks a little like a footballer kicking with the inside of the foot. As this is the first time you have had one foot in the air for any length of time, it provides an excellent test of your balance – and performed slowly, of course, for the duration of one whole in-breath.

Look for the feeling of energy between right palm and left forearm

Your elbows should be lower than your wrists

Really sink your weight into your right leg as you go back

Ex**hale**

90%

The toes of your right foot are turned outwards, with the sole parallel to the ground

In**hale**

100%

2 Place your right foot down behind again, in what feels almost like a gentle rocking movement. Make contact with the toes first, not the heel or sole. Empty the weight from your left foot, then draw your left heel across and place it down in a narrow stance ahead of your right foot. Simultaneously, your arms move into the typical Play Guitar configuration, but this time with your left arm extended forwards and the palm of your right hand facing inwards towards your left forearm.

Brush Knee and Push

Once again, this is a repetition of a movement you have already learned, with just one difference: this time you are approaching it from a narrow heel stance (Play Guitar), whereas before it was from a narrow toe stance (Crane Spreads its Wings, see page 56).

BEGIN BY letting go of the Play Guitar shape in your arms and rotating your waist clockwise.

1 Draw your right palm back behind you, just as you did with the movement on page 57. Again, try to keep your gaze on the palm as it drifts back, but without turning your head too much. Ideally, your chin should remain in line with your breastbone and navel. Think of holding something tangible in your palm, which is facing upwards at this stage.

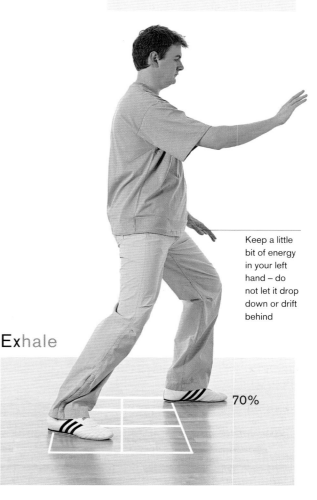

Keep a little bit of energy in your left hand – do not let it drop down or drift behind

Exhale

70%

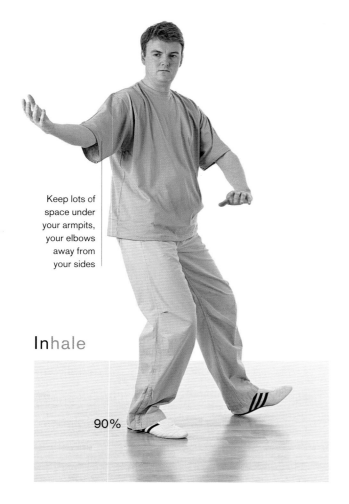

Keep lots of space under your armpits, your elbows away from your sides

Inhale

90%

2 Turn your waist back now, counter-clockwise, and step out wide and slightly forwards with your left foot. Brush your left knee with your left palm as before (see page 57), and then rotate your right palm and push out, straight ahead as your left knee bends and the weight goes forward. Your gaze is now directed outwards as if towards a distant horizon.

Step Forward, Parry and Punch

Next comes a lengthy, forward-stepping sequence that reminds us of tai chi's martial origins with a punch at the end! Despite this, you should not suddenly speed up and become tense. Think of the fist as being simply a symbol of your individual will and determination, not of aggression in any sense.

BEGIN BY shifting your weight back into your right leg and forming a loose fist with your right hand.

1 Raise the toes of your left foot and pivot on the heel to point the foot outwards. At the same time, allow your right hand, with its loose fist, to slide over and down, left of centre, to about hip height. Meanwhile, your left arm has straightened somewhat so that the fingers are pointing downwards, adjacent to but not in contact with your left thigh.

2 Flatten your left foot, then step ahead with your right foot, placing it down with the toes pointing outwards. As you step, allow your right hand, still in a loose fist, to circle over and down to a position just above your right hip, rotating as it goes so that the knuckle side of the hand is turned towards the ground. Your left palm follows a little, to settle at your centre.

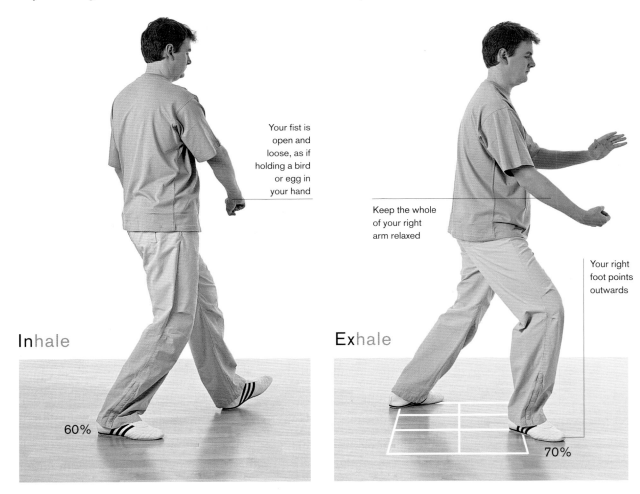

Your fist is open and loose, as if holding a bird or egg in your hand

Keep the whole of your right arm relaxed

Your right foot points outwards

Inhale

60%

Exhale

70%

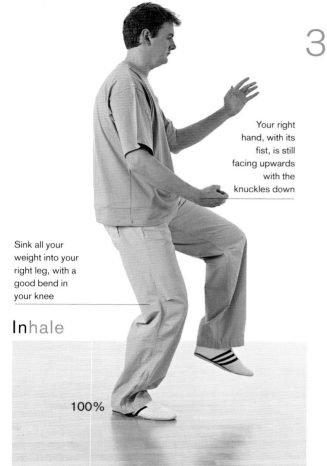

3 Lift your left foot from the ground and prepare to step straight ahead by drawing in the toes just a little towards your right heel. Turn your waist slightly clockwise as you draw back your right hand, knuckles still facing downwards. At the same time, your left forearm starts to rise to a near-vertical position at your centre. All this is in preparation for the final movement – the parry and 'punch' itself.

Your right hand, with its fist, is still facing upwards with the knuckles down

Sink all your weight into your right leg, with a good bend in your knee

Inhale

100%

Keep a little softness in your elbow, even at the end of the movement, so that it is not fully extended

Adjust the back heel to a comfortable position as your weight goes forward

Exhale

70%

4 Step ahead with your left foot and bend your knee as the weight goes forward. At the same time, sweep your left forearm across to the left, away from your centre, then project your right hand forward in the 'punch'. Do this by simply unbending your right elbow. Your right hand rotates in mid-flight, to finish with the thumb-side uppermost. You may find it helpful to count aloud while learning the steps of this exercise: 'one, two and three', finishing with the punch.

Release Arm and Push

This part of the sequence is especially good for promoting flexibility in your wrists and elbow joints. It takes a while to master, but is well worth the effort. It is interesting to note just how much of the movement comes from the turning of your waist, first slightly counter-clockwise, then clockwise, and finally returning to centre.

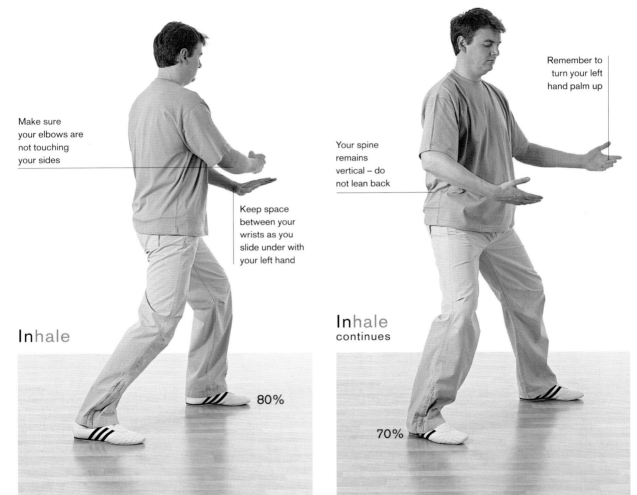

Make sure your elbows are not touching your sides

Keep space between your wrists as you slide under with your left hand

Inhale

80%

Remember to turn your left hand palm up

Your spine remains vertical – do not lean back

Inhale continues

70%

BEGIN BY relaxing your arms and turning your waist just a little counter-clockwise.

1 Draw your right hand, still in a fist, across to a position left of centre with your forearm more or less horizontal. Then slide your left hand beneath your right forearm and beyond, the fingers pointing forwards and the palm facing downwards for the moment.

2 Now let go of the fist and rotate both hands to a palms-up position. Then shift your weight back and rotate your waist clockwise, while simultaneously drawing your right hand back across your left forearm. This appears to 'release' your right arm and set it free from the left, but the expansive character of the movement is actually achieved by the action of your waist and the shifting of your weight to the back leg.

3 Prepare to push out by turning both palms to face forwards and rotating your centre to face straight ahead also. The push that concludes this movement is similar to the one described on page 50, except that here the left foot is placed forward instead of the right. So, simply return your weight to your left foot by bending your knee and make the push shape with your hands.

BENEFITS

• Rotations of the wrist have their origin at the elbow, so this movement will retain the suppleness and strength of this joint and help avoid problems like 'tennis elbow'.

• The intricacy of the movement will also improve your dexterity and co-ordination.

Do not thrust forward with your palms – just use the bend of your knee to create the 'push'

Do not lean into your push. Keep the back straight

Front knee just above the toes – no further!

Exhale

70%

Turn and Close part 1

Traditionally, the Short Yang Form comes in two parts. You are now at the end of part 1 and have completed around 2 minutes of tai chi movement – no mean achievement. In fact, many of the benefits of tai chi can be gained simply by sticking to part 1, repeating it several times to make up a 10-minute spell of activity.

BENEFITS

• This movement exercises and stimulates the muscles and ligaments of the shoulders.

• It provides further movement around the areas of vital lymphatic tissue centred in the neck, chest and armpits.

• The closing movement is also deeply relaxing — breathe calmly and deeply to find that special place of inner stillness.

BEGIN BY transferring a good percentage of your weight into your right leg.

1 Relax your hands and begin to pivot slowly on your left heel to help turn your waist clockwise, returning in a moment to face your original opening direction. The aspect of your hands here is initially rather like somebody warming their hands at a fire, palms forward and facing slightly downwards, but as you turn they begin to lift a little and separate out from each other.

Your hands are relaxed, gliding gently apart

Sink back into the right foot

Inhale

90%

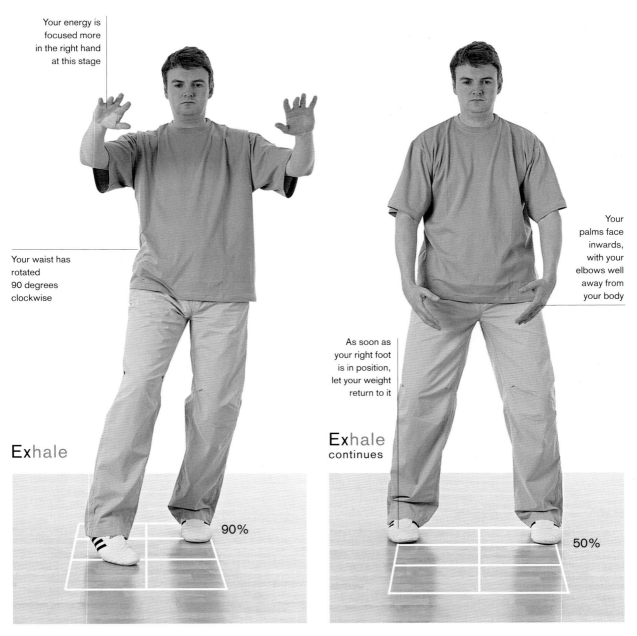

Your energy is focused more in the right hand at this stage

Your waist has rotated 90 degrees clockwise

Your palms face inwards, with your elbows well away from your body

As soon as your right foot is in position, let your weight return to it

Exhale

Exhale
continues

90%

50%

2 Transfer your weight back into your left side and rotate your body clockwise 90 degrees. Allow your hands to continue separating, forming an ever-widening arc that in a moment will become a full circle. Then raise your right heel and begin drawing back your right foot into a position parallel with your left.

3 Your hands continue on their circular journey, down and then inwards once more, to meet (without touching) in front of your lower abdomen. Return half your weight into your right side now, making for a rare 50/50 stance, similar to that at the start (see page 42). Your palms should be facing inwards at this stage, the fingers relaxed.

4 With the next in-breath, your hands begin to rise together, palms inward-facing, up through your centre until they cross, your left wrist resting for a moment very lightly upon the right at about chin height. Your left forearm is therefore closer to you than the right as your wrists cross.

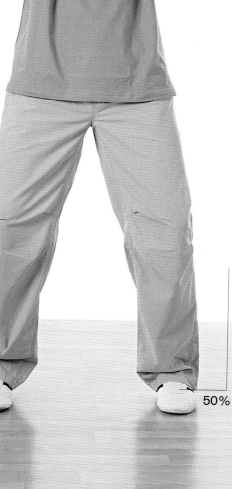

Keep your shoulders relaxed as you raise your arms

Keep the knees soft, even as the arms rise

Feet parallel to each other, shoulder-width apart

50%

Inhale

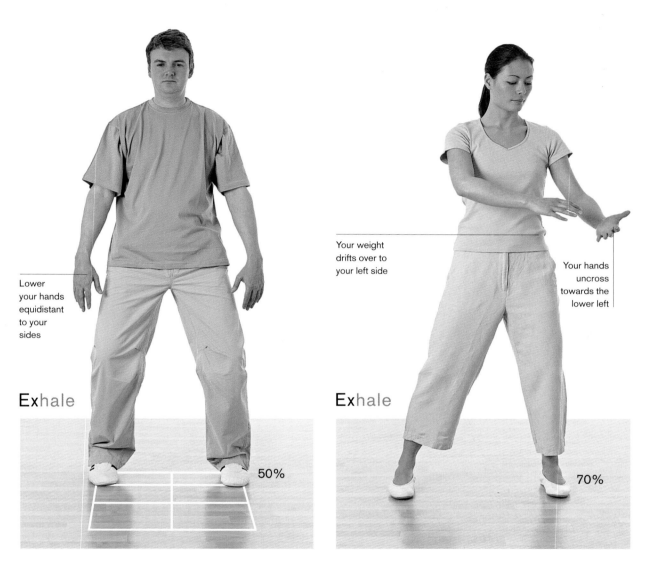

Lower
your hands
equidistant
to your
sides

Your weight
drifts over to
your left side

Your hands
uncross
towards the
lower left

Exhale

Exhale

50%

70%

5 **TO FINISH**, simply lower your arms gently down
through your centre, allowing them to separate
naturally as they fall to your sides. Sink down a little as
you exhale. This is a traditional closing movement and
you can finish your tai chi session at this point.

6 **OR TO GO ON TO PART 2.** Here, the weight will
flow a little more into your left side as you lower the
arms, and your hands will be drawn down left of
centre, as they fall, with the left palm beginning to turn
up in readiness for the next movement, which will
commence part 2.

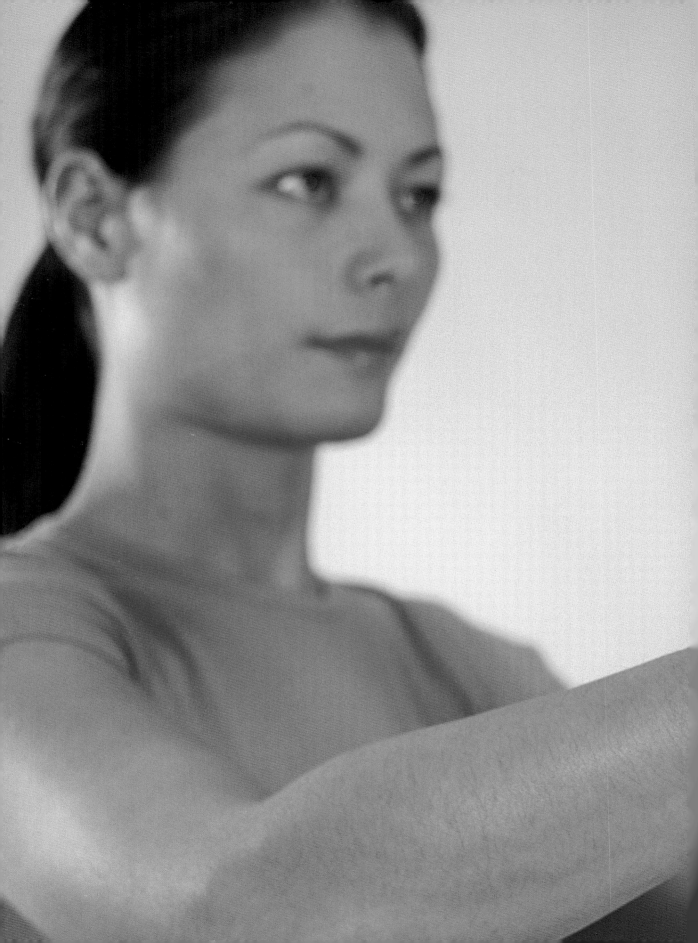

the
short yang
form

Carry Tiger to Mountain

This is the first time we encounter diagonal steps. Carry Tiger involves a large, 135-degree turn to a point behind your right shoulder. If you think of the compass, and your starting point as facing south, then this movement is heading north-west – the direction of The Mountain in ancient Chinese philosophy.

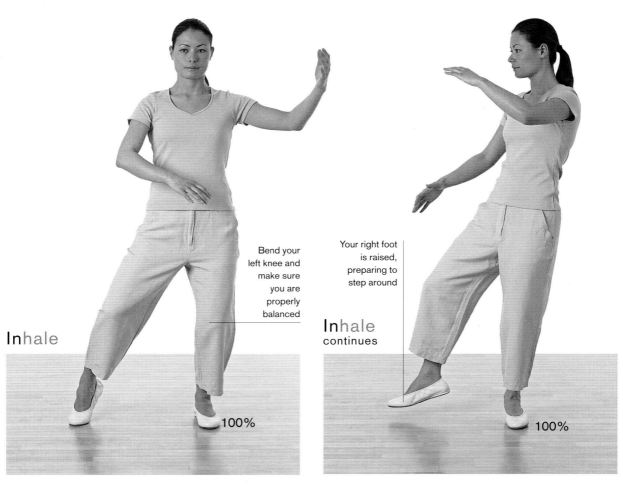

Bend your left knee and make sure you are properly balanced

Inhale

100%

Your right foot is raised, preparing to step around

Inhale
continues

100%

BEGIN BY referring to the alternative position 6 at the conclusion of the previous movement (see page 67), with much of your weight already transferred to your left foot.

1 With your right arm still across your centre, separate your hands by raising your left arm a little with the palm facing upwards. Lift your right heel from the ground and draw the toes in towards your left foot to test your balance. This is all about preparing for the large turn you are about to make on to the diagonal behind.

2 Open up your right hip and rotate your waist clockwise way around to your right, then begin to place your foot down on the diagonal behind your right shoulder. It takes practice before you can achieve this big step around, so don't despair if you cannot manage the whole thing first time. The secret lies in really sinking down into your left side before committing yourself to the turn.

3 As you place your right foot down, make sure it is with the heel first, and then bend your knee. As this is a very large step around, it is more important than ever to adjust your back foot to a comfortable position at the end. Meanwhile, your right hand sweeps across your right knee as you go, to eventually turn palm up, as if supporting a large ball, with your left hand on top.

Right palm turns up at the conclusion of the turn

Front knee just above the toes – no further!

Pivot on your back heel to a comfortable position as soon as possible

Exhale

70%

Diagonal Rollback and Press

The diagonal Chorus (see pages 38–39) begins here. You are already facing the diagonal, of course, so all you need to do here is sit back into your left foot and turn your waist first counter-clockwise, then clockwise as you progress through the movements.

BEGIN BY rotating your waist a little clockwise and shifting your weight back slowly into your left side.

1 With your front foot still resting in place on the diagonal, rotate or 'roll' your hands slightly while sliding your left palm, at a distance, down your right forearm to a position just beside your elbow. Meanwhile, the angle of your right elbow has become more acute, so that the forearm is almost pointing upwards. During all this, rotate your waist slightly clockwise, with your arms following slightly to the right as well.

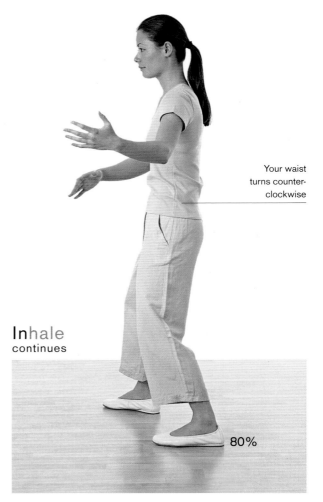

Your waist turns counter-clockwise

Inhale
continues

80%

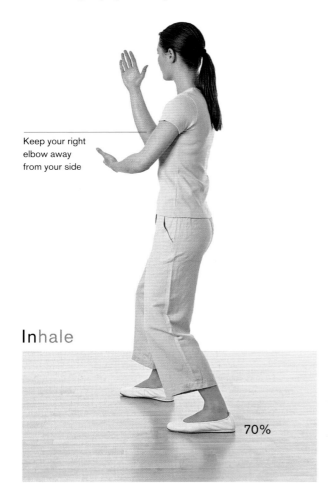

Keep your right elbow away from your side

Inhale

70%

2 Still with your inhalation, rotate your waist counter-clockwise and draw your left hand back and around towards your left hip, while your right forearm folds down across your centre. Most of your weight is now in your back leg. Try to cultivate a feeling of contact between your palms even though they remain separated – keep thinking of that energetic connection between your hands.

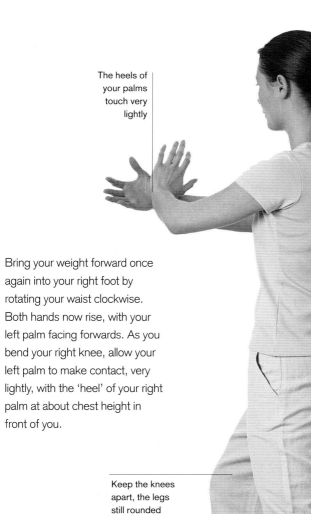

The heels of your palms touch very lightly

BENEFITS

• The diagonal Chorus further assists in developing proper alignment of the hips and shoulders with the spine.

• It also makes you more aware of your orientation and personal space, through challenging changes of direction and footwork.

3 Bring your weight forward once again into your right foot by rotating your waist clockwise. Both hands now rise, with your left palm facing forwards. As you bend your right knee, allow your left palm to make contact, very lightly, with the 'heel' of your right palm at about chest height in front of you.

Keep the knees apart, the legs still rounded and arch-like

Exhale

70%

Diagonal Separate Hands and Push

Still facing that diagonal, and keeping your feet flat on the ground, you now go through the routine you learned on page 50 – but make sure your feet are correctly placed. This is the challenge with any wide stance on a diagonal axis. If you feel awkward at any stage, your stance is almost certainly too narrow.

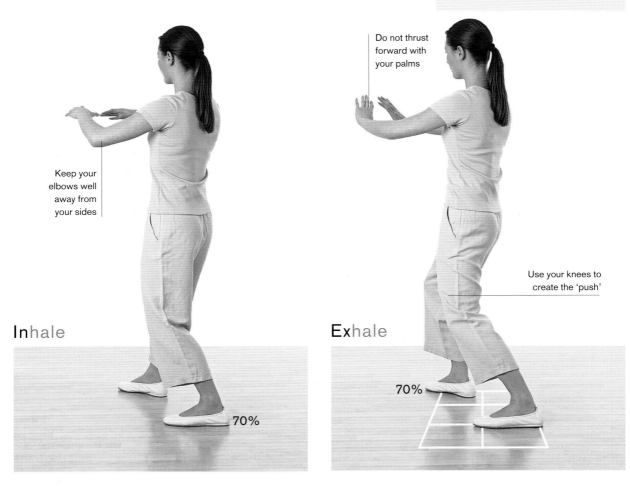

Keep your elbows well away from your sides

Do not thrust forward with your palms

Use your knees to create the 'push'

Inhale

70%

Exhale

70%

BEGIN BY letting go of the previous formation of your hands and rolling your palms into a downward-facing position.

1 Separate your hands horizontally with a little 'swimming' motion, outwards and back, with your thumbs pointing towards your chest. At the same time, transfer your weight into your back foot. A common error at this point is to lean backwards, as if recoiling in shock. Whenever you suspect that you might be leaning, sink downwards instead.

2 Rotate your hands so that the palms are facing outwards, then bring your weight forward once again by bending your right knee. Your shoulders and arms do not travel any great distance during this. The appearance of the 'push' comes from the hands and is made by bending your knees, not thrusting forward with your arms. Remember not to lean into the push: keep in mind the internal plumb line (see page 29), and keep your back straight throughout. As you exhale, let go mentally of any tension in your chest.

Diagonal Single Whip

It's now time for the Single Whip once again. The big difference here, of course, is that the whole sequence starts and finishes on the diagonal axis. You will need to make sure you are fully balanced and comfortable in your weighted (right) foot before commencing the final big 180-degree manoeuvre around to the left.

BEGIN BY shifting most of your weight into your back leg and allowing your arms to relax.

1 Your hands flatten with palms down, and you should find that your arms extend naturally without effort as you straighten your right knee. Just sit back and relax into the movement. Keep your elbows soft, with a little 'give' in your arms at all times.

2 Keeping your arms in the same outstretched position, slowly rotate your centre counter-clockwise by pivoting on your right heel. Your feet should become slightly 'pigeon-toed' – as if placed on the sides of a triangle. At the end of this turn, both feet should be flat on the ground, with the weight mostly in your left side.

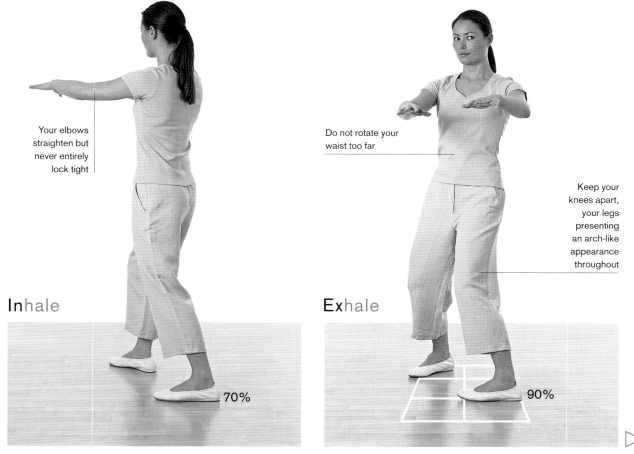

Your elbows straighten but never entirely lock tight

Do not rotate your waist too far

Keep your knees apart, your legs presenting an arch-like appearance throughout

Inhale

Exhale

70%

90%

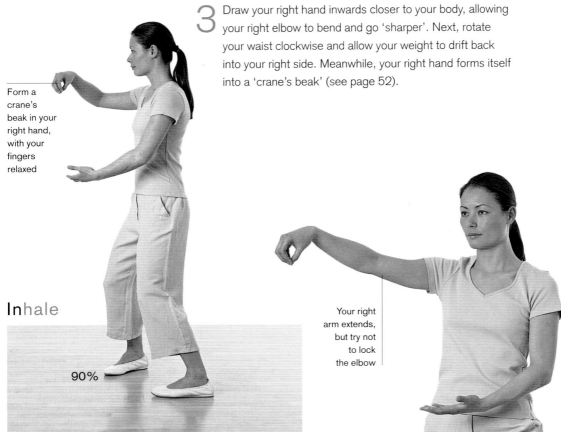

3 Draw your right hand inwards closer to your body, allowing your right elbow to bend and go 'sharper'. Next, rotate your waist clockwise and allow your weight to drift back into your right side. Meanwhile, your right hand forms itself into a 'crane's beak' (see page 52).

Form a crane's beak in your right hand, with your fingers relaxed

Inhale

90%

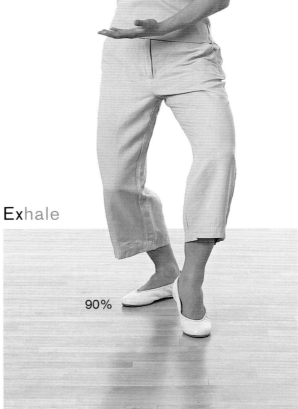

Your right arm extends, but try not to lock the elbow

Exhale

90%

4 Project your crane's beak outwards, just right of centre, until your arm is almost straight. At the same time, pivot on the toes of your left foot and rotate your centre counter-clockwise. Try to keep your chin in line with your breastbone and navel. Your weight remains predominantly in your right foot, allowing the toes of your left foot to pivot freely.

5 Sink all your weight into your right foot, preparing to step around to your far left. This is a big step, so make sure your balance is established before you raise your left foot from the ground. By this time, your left hand has already begun to rise from its position close to your right hip.

A good bend in your right knee helps you balance

Inhale

100%

Make sure your feet are still shoulder-width apart

Exhale

6 Step right around on to the diagonal, making contact with your left heel first and then bending your left knee as your weight settles forward. Your left hand rises and rotates as you go, to finish with the palm and fingers facing straight ahead, in front of your left breast, with your elbow relaxed. Meanwhile, your right arm remains extended and slightly behind you, the crane's beak still intact.

70%

Fist Under Elbow

After our series of repetitions, it is now time to learn some new movements and also return for a while to the square axis. The fist appears once again here, but as before (see page 60) the shape is a loose, relaxed formation. Again, if it helps, try counting aloud 'one, two and three' during this routine.

BEGIN BY opening up your hands in a relaxed fashion and shifting your weight back into your right leg.

Try not to let your left arm drift away too far to the side

1 Pivot on your left heel, to turn your foot outwards a little. This will take you back onto the regular square axis that you used in Part 1. Allow your waist to rotate a little with your foot, so slightly counter-clockwise. If you wish, count aloud the number 'one' at this point.

Your waist rotates counter-clockwise as you pivot on your left heel

Inhale

90%

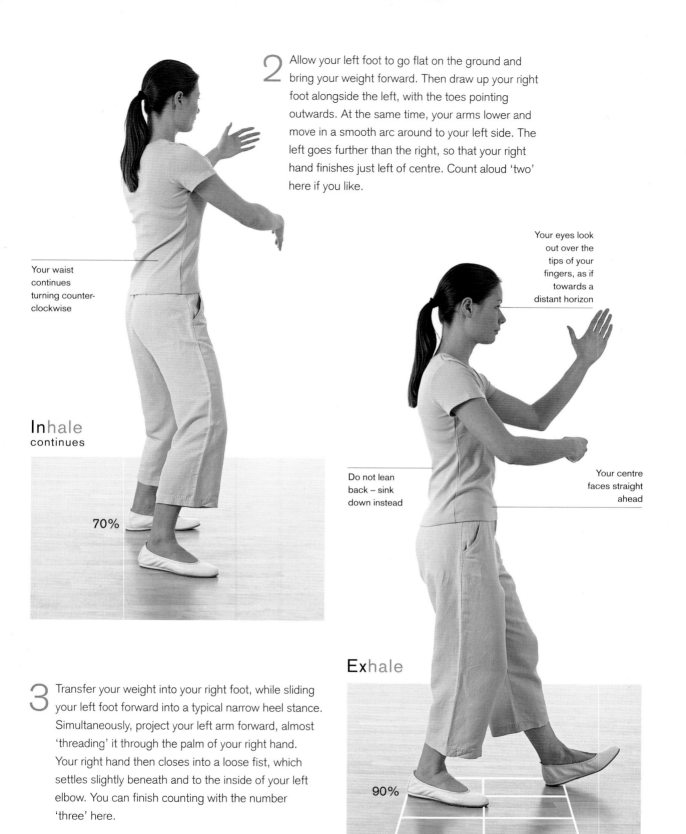

2 Allow your left foot to go flat on the ground and bring your weight forward. Then draw up your right foot alongside the left, with the toes pointing outwards. At the same time, your arms lower and move in a smooth arc around to your left side. The left goes further than the right, so that your right hand finishes just left of centre. Count aloud 'two' here if you like.

Your waist continues turning counter-clockwise

Your eyes look out over the tips of your fingers, as if towards a distant horizon

Inhale
continues

Do not lean back – sink down instead

Your centre faces straight ahead

70%

Exhale

3 Transfer your weight into your right foot, while sliding your left foot forward into a typical narrow heel stance. Simultaneously, project your left arm forward, almost 'threading' it through the palm of your right hand. Your right hand then closes into a loose fist, which settles slightly beneath and to the inside of your left elbow. You can finish counting with the number 'three' here.

90%

Repulse Monkey, right

This sequence mimics the movement of the monkey, with long, swinging arms and swaying hips. It presents us with backward steps for the first time, and is repeated here three times. Each movement concludes with a flourish of the palm, pushing out – first with the right palm, then the left, and finally the right palm again.

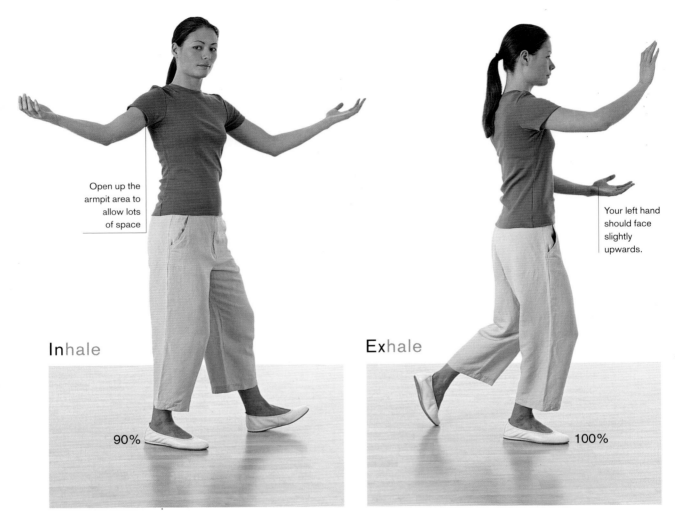

Open up the armpit area to allow lots of space

Your left hand should face slightly upwards.

Inhale

90%

Exhale

100%

BEGIN BY letting go of the fist in your right hand and turning your left palm upwards.

1 Rotate your waist clockwise and circle back with your right palm while keeping most of the weight in your back leg. Your palm rises to about the height of your chin, no further. Allow your eyes to follow your right hand as it goes.

2 Lift your left foot and draw it back behind you. You are in the process of stepping back with your left foot. At the same time, start to lower your left hand, so that the palm falls towards the level of your waist, left of centre. Meanwhile, your right palm rotates to face forwards, in preparation for the push that is to come.

BENEFITS

• This exercise makes you aware of the space behind you, where you cannot see, and promotes fluent movement in an unfamiliar direction.

• Mastering such movements will make you stronger mentally and emotionally.

• These steps also increase muscle tone in your upper arms and shoulders.

3 Making contact with your toes first, place the whole of your left foot down behind you, flat on the ground, and move your weight into it. Your right palm pushes forward as you sink into your left side, while your left hand settles at waist height, left of centre. Finally, adjust your right foot by pivoting on your right heel so that the toes face forwards.

Avoid tension in your right wrist as you show your palm

Your elbow is lower than your hand and not tight

Exhale
continues

Both feet are flat on the ground

90%

Repulse Monkey, left

This movement is very similar to the previous one, but performed on the opposite side. This time you start with your right foot and right palm forward, and the sequence opens with your feet flat on the ground instead of the narrow heel stance of before (see page 80).

BEGIN BY relaxing your right arm and rotating your wrist to turn your palm upwards.

1 Rotate your waist counter-clockwise and circle back with your left palm while keeping most of your weight in the back leg. Your palm rises to about the height of your chin, no further. Allow your eyes to follow your left hand as it goes.

Make sure there is space between your elbows and your sides

Make contact with your toes first

Exhale

100%

Do not turn your waist until you have turned your right palm upwards

Inhale

90%

2 Lift your right foot and draw it back. You are in the process of stepping backwards with your right foot. At the same time, start to lower your right hand, so that the palm falls towards the level of your waist, right of centre. Meanwhile, your left palm begins to rotate to face forwards, in preparation for the push that is to come.

BENEFITS

• This movement opens up and gently stimulates the areas in the chest, throat, armpits and groin associated with the lymphatic system (see page 19).

• It also helps to improve muscle tone in your calves.

3 Making contact with your toes first, place the whole of your right foot down flat on the ground and move your weight into it. Your left palm pushes forwards as you sink into your right side, while your right hand settles at about waist height, right of centre. Finally, adjust your left foot by pivoting on your left heel so that the toes face forwards.

Both feet are flat on the ground

Exhale
continues

90%

Repulse Monkey, right

To conclude the full Repulse Monkey sequence, you repeat the right-sided version met with already on pages 80–81. We show it again in full, however, as the starting position is just a little different this time.

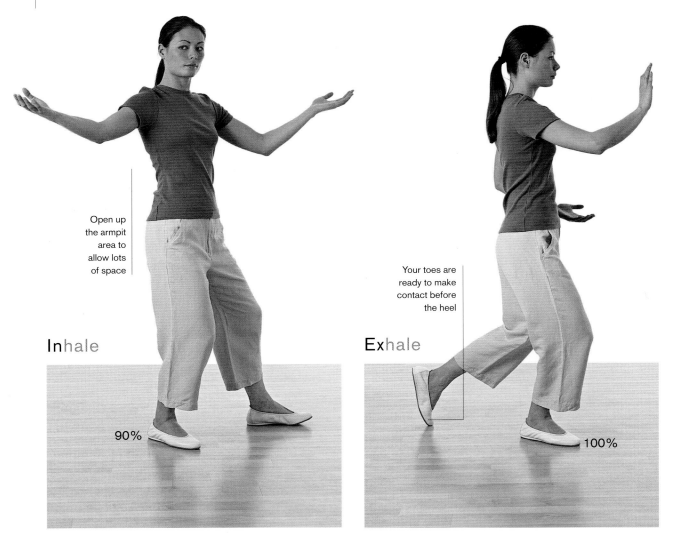

Open up the armpit area to allow lots of space

Inhale

90%

Your toes are ready to make contact before the heel

Exhale

100%

BEGIN BY relaxing your left arm and turning your left palm upwards.

1 Rotate your waist clockwise and circle back with your right palm while keeping most of the weight in your back leg. Your palm rises to about the height of your chin, no further. Allow your eyes to follow your right hand as it goes.

2 Lift your left foot and draw it back behind you. You are in the process of stepping back with your left foot. At the same time, start to lower your left hand, so that the palm falls towards the level of your waist, left of centre. Meanwhile, your right palm rotates to face forwards, in preparation for the push that is to come.

BENEFITS

• As before (see pages 80–81), this exercise helps you to master backward movements, and strengthens will-power and self-confidence.

• It also increases muscle tone in your upper arms and shoulders.

• Repeating the steps further increases your sense of co-ordination and balance.

Keep plenty of space between your left elbow and your side

3 Making contact with your toes first, place the whole of your left foot down flat on the ground and move your weight into it. Your right palm pushes forward as you sink into your left side, while your left hand settles at waist height, left of centre. Finally, adjust your right foot by pivoting on your right heel so that the toes face forwards.

Both feet are flat on the ground

Exhale
continues

90%

Diagonal Flying

Sometimes called 'Slant Flying', this movement requires a 135-degree turn of your body to settle on to the diagonal axis, way around behind your right shoulder. The dynamic flourish at the end provides you with a good sense of closure to the Repulse Monkey sequence that precedes it – as if putting the monkey back on the tree.

BEGIN BY rotating your waist a little counter-clockwise and allowing your right heel to follow.

1 Form a ball with your hands, just left of centre. Your left hand is on top of the ball, palm down, while your right hand supports the ball from underneath, palm up. Sink well down into your left foot, ready for the big step around that comes next.

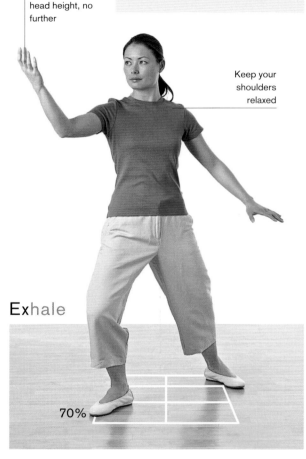

Your right hand rises to about head height, no further

Keep your shoulders relaxed

Exhale

70%

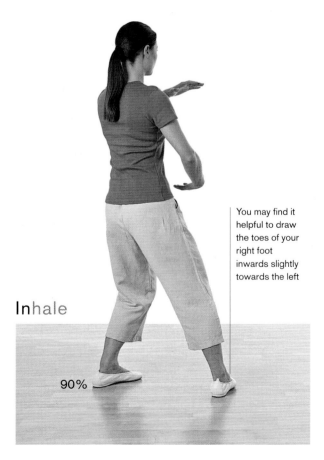

You may find it helpful to draw the toes of your right foot inwards slightly towards the left

Inhale

90%

2 With your right foot raised, direct your waist around clockwise and place your right foot down, heel first on to the diagonal behind your right shoulder. Your arms open up as you go, with your right arm sweeping upwards in a great arc, right of centre, while your left hand drops to the level of your left hip, palm down and facing backwards slightly. It is important to adjust your back foot to a comfortable position as soon as possible.

Cloudy Hands, opening

The Cloudy Hands sequence focuses on sideways stepping and involves plenty of rotations of your waist, the steps themselves progressing from right to left each time. To get started, you have to position yourself back on to the square axis, which is the purpose of the next short movement.

BEGIN BY rotating your waist clockwise and bringing all your weight forward into your right foot.

1 Draw up your left foot in line with your right, so that your feet are now side by side but at least one-and-a-half shoulder widths apart. At the same time, sweep your left hand around close to your right hip, the palm turning up to support a ball from beneath, while your right hand rolls over to rest on top of the ball.

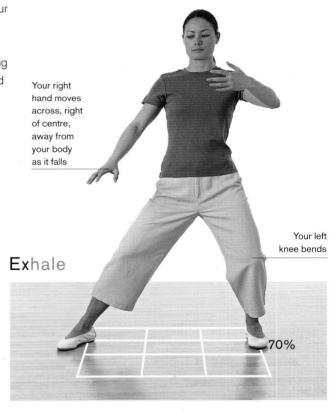

Your right hand moves across, right of centre, away from your body as it falls

Your left knee bends

Exhale

70%

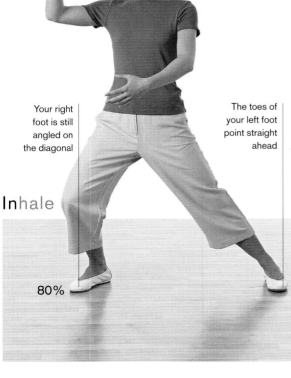

Your right foot is still angled on the diagonal

The toes of your left foot point straight ahead

Inhale

80%

2 Shift your weight across into your left side and change your hands, so that your right hand drops to about hip height while the left rises to about throat height. Your left hand rises inside your right – in other words, it is closer to your body than the right. Try to make the movements soft and curvaceous rather than just up and down.

Cloudy Hands, left

You are now beginning the sideways-stepping routine that characterizes Cloudy Hands proper. Your legs and feet remain parallel as you step in a 'plodding' movement, with your knees bent like a great arch and very strong. The hands, however, remain soft, as if describing the shapes of billowing clouds in the air.

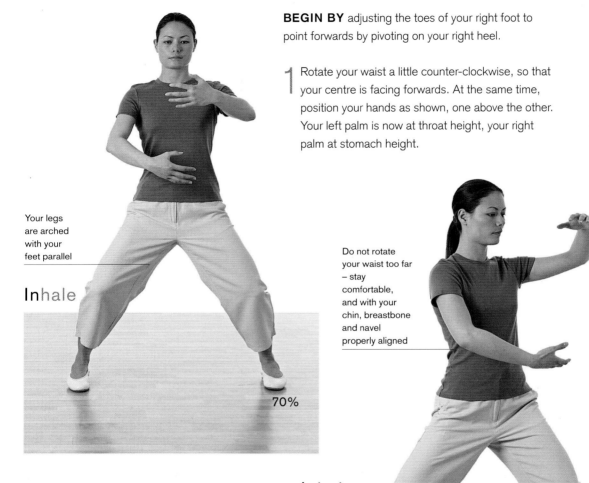

BEGIN BY adjusting the toes of your right foot to point forwards by pivoting on your right heel.

1 Rotate your waist a little counter-clockwise, so that your centre is facing forwards. At the same time, position your hands as shown, one above the other. Your left palm is now at throat height, your right palm at stomach height.

Your legs are arched with your feet parallel

Inhale

70%

Do not rotate your waist too far – stay comfortable, and with your chin, breastbone and navel properly aligned

Inhale
continues

90%

2 Rotating your waist still further in a counter-clockwise direction, form a ball with your hands, left hand on top – so your wrists rotate slightly as you turn. Keep a good distance between your arms and your body – 30 cm (12 in) is about right, depending on your proportions and height.

3 With your weight now in your left side, lift and draw your right foot inwards to about shoulder width from your left, still parallel with your left foot and with the toes pointing forwards. Then change hands, by lowering the left and raising the right. Your upper arm extends slightly further to your left to make space for the lower one to rise inside of it, closer to your body. At this point your weight shifts across slightly into your right side.

BENEFITS

• The constant turning of the waist in these movements benefits your digestive system.

• Over time, it can add greater muscle tone to your waistline, and also gradually increases flexibility.

Make sure the knees stay well apart

Your feet should still be no closer to each other than the width of your shoulders

Exhale

60%

Cloudy Hands, right

This sequence is almost the same as the steps on pages 88–89. It is only the starting position that is a little different, with your feet positioned much closer together and parallel. As you step from right to left, think of a 'plodding' motion, keeping your knees apart and planting your feet down perfectly flat each time.

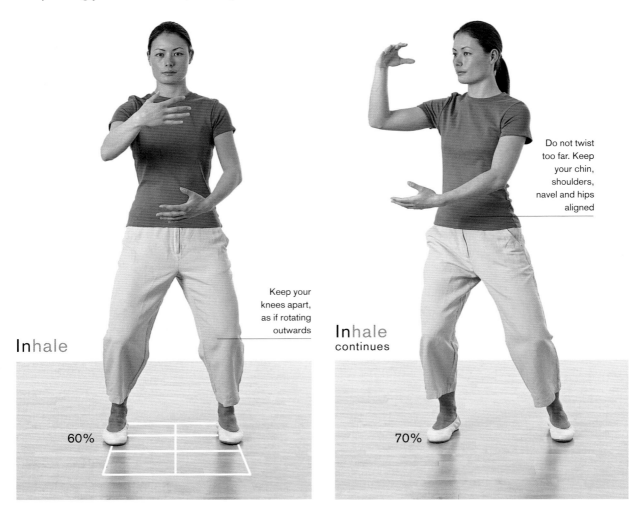

Keep your knees apart, as if rotating outwards

Inhale

60%

Do not twist too far. Keep your chin, shoulders, navel and hips aligned

Inhale continues

70%

BEGIN BY rotating your waist clockwise, to face forwards once again.

1 With your centre now directed straight ahead, position your hands as shown, one above the other. Your right palm is at throat height, your left palm at stomach height. Visualize your whole spinal column rotating with these subtle turns of your waist, keeping your head, shoulders and hips squared up throughout.

2 Slowly turn your waist clockwise and, equally slowly, rotate your wrists to form a ball, with your right hand on top. Do not turn too far. As always, your bottom should remain tucked in, not jutting out, and your knees retain plenty of space between them, remaining arch-like through the entire sequence.

BENEFITS

• The movements of the whole Cloudy Hands sequence have a particularly calming effect on the emotions.

• They also help build softness and relaxation in your hands and even your fingers.

3 Step along to the left with your left foot to a distance of one-and-a-half shoulder widths from your right foot, then change your hands so that the right drops to about hip height while the left rises to about throat height. Your left hand rises inside your right, while your upper arm extends slightly further to your right to make space for the lower one to rise inside it, closer to your body.

Shift your weight into your left side just before your right hand comes down

Exhale

70%

Cloudy Hands, left into Whip

As you may have realized, you could continue happily with the Cloudy Hands routine indefinitely, stepping sideways from right to left forever. But at this point we will conclude the sequence with a clever half-step forward into the final stages of a Single Whip.

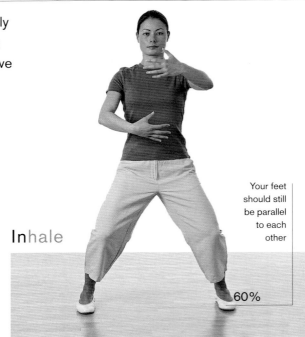

Inhale

Your feet should still be parallel to each other

60%

BEGIN BY turning your centre counter-clockwise to face forwards once again.

1 As before, position your hands as shown, with the left hand above the right. Your left hand is at about throat height, your right at about stomach height, with a generous distance between your arms and your body. Your feet are wide apart again and your legs arched.

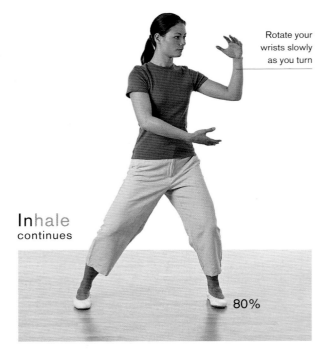

Rotate your wrists slowly as you turn

Inhale
continues

80%

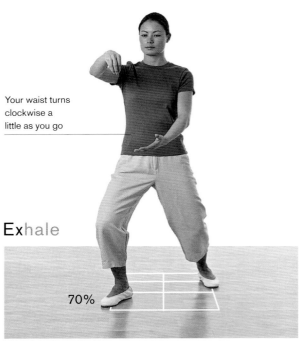

Your waist turns clockwise a little as you go

Exhale

70%

2 Rotate your waist counter-clockwise again and form a ball with your hands, left hand on top. Try to establish a smooth, rotational flow to your wrist movement. We have to show them 'frozen in time' in the photographs, but remember that in practice there is always movement and change at the heart of all tai chi technique.

3 Now for something different. As you change hands this time, step forward one half-pace with your right heel and shift your weight forward by bending your knee. Your right hand rises in the form of a crane's beak (see page 52) as your left palm follows around to settle underneath, close to your right hip.

Isolated Single Whip

You are now about to break into the middle stages of the Single Whip (see page 51). It is called 'Isolated' here because this is the only time it occurs outside the Chorus. What comes next, therefore, is just the concluding part of the Single Whip – the one in-breath and one out-breath as you step around to the right.

BEGIN BY emptying all your weight from your left leg.

1 Prepare to step around to your left by drawing the toes of your left foot inwards a little closer to your right foot, ready for the turn. As always, this is to test your balance. As you commence your step, your left arm begins to rise and your hand alters from a palm-up position to one in which the palm is beginning to face inwards.

2 Continue rotating your waist counter-clockwise and complete the step around 90 degrees with your left foot into a wide stance, making contact with the heel first before bending your knee. As soon as the weight returns to your left side, adjust the back foot to a comfortable position by pivoting on your right heel. Your left hand has now rotated to point fingers ahead, with the elbow rounded and soft.

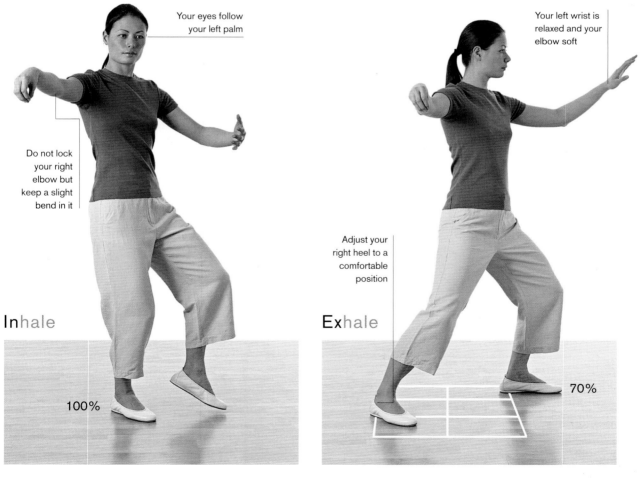

Your eyes follow your left palm

Do not lock your right elbow but keep a slight bend in it

Inhale

100%

Your left wrist is relaxed and your elbow soft

Adjust your right heel to a comfortable position

Exhale

70%

Snake Creeps Down

This is a classic move, and the first of those involving upward and downward energies. It can really test the flexibility of your hips and knees, but there is no need to strive to be super-flexible. The photographs show a gentle version, without too great a stretch, which is perfectly adequate for our purpose.

BEGIN BY relaxing your left hand and bringing most of your weight temporarily forward into your left foot.

1 Lengthen your stance by shuffling or sliding back (this depends on the surface on which you are working) with your right foot. Then return your weight to your right foot, rotate your waist clockwise and begin to bend your right knee, to 'squat' down on the back leg. Meanwhile, your left palm traces back to a position roughly facing your chest.

• This movement vigorously exercises the joints of the hips, knees and ankles.

• It stimulates and gently tones the muscles of the upper thigh and buttocks.

• It also disperses stagnant energies in the area of the Liver and Gall Bladder, located in the lower right side. Imagine brushing away any frustration or anger with your left hand.

The crane's beak remains intact

Your right knee should be directly over your foot for stability

Inhale

90%

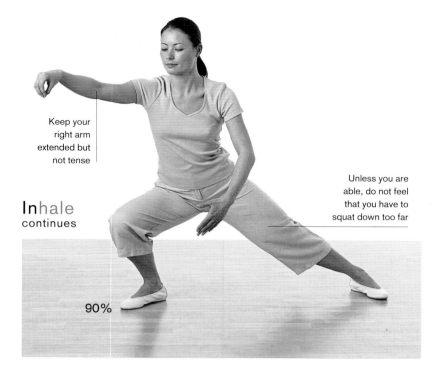

Keep your right arm extended but not tense

Inhale continues

Unless you are able, do not feel that you have to squat down too far

90%

2 Pivot a little on your left heel if you can, to point your toes inwards as you continue to sink down and squat on your right knee. Your waist continues to rotate clockwise, and your left hand has now progressed right down in a graceful arc to a position close to your right leg.

3 Your left hand now continues its journey by thrusting forward, close to the ground, as you realign your front foot by pointing the toes straight ahead again. If you were to trace its path through the air, you would find that your left hand roughly describes a large clockwise circle back, down and forward during this movement.

Your left foot straightens once more

Exhale

90%

Golden Pheasant Stands on Left Leg

In contrast to the previous movement, which was low-slung and mysterious, here everything is upright and very much 'up front'. This is the cock bird showing off, strutting on one leg – you have to raise your right leg off the ground and keep it there for a second or two, so prepare carefully and be sure of your balance first.

BENEFITS

• This movement helps develop your balance and self-confidence.

• It strengthens the bones of your legs, assisting you to avoid illnesses such as osteoporosis.

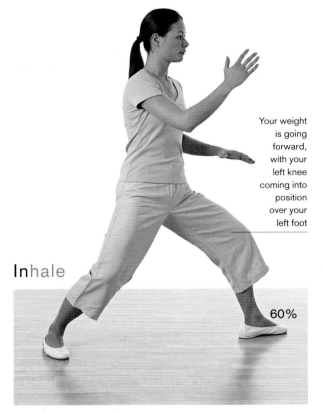

Your weight is going forward, with your left knee coming into position over your left foot

Inhale

60%

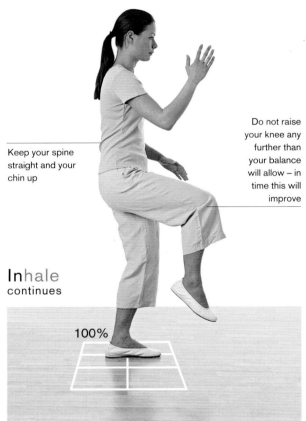

Keep your spine straight and your chin up

Do not raise your knee any further than your balance will allow – in time this will improve

Inhale continues

100%

BEGIN BY extricating yourself from the squat. This means raising your body and bringing your weight forward, and there is a precise way of doing this.

1 Pivot on your back heel to turn your toes inwards a little, then adjust your front foot by turning the toes outwards, again by pivoting on the heel. All this is in preparation for the next movement, which requires a stable base from which your body can go forward and up. In the photograph, this has already started to take place and the arms have moved forward and up.

2 The major part of this movement is unusual as it accompanies the in-breath. Still with the inhalation, bring all your weight into your left foot and then raise your right knee to finish beneath your right elbow. In fact, your forearm, elbow, knee and shin should all finish in one vertical plane, not sticking out to one side or the other.

Golden Pheasant Stands on Right Leg

The previous movement is now repeated on the opposite side. Until now, you have always had at least the tip of a toe or a convenient heel on the ground most of the time. Now the 'stabilizers' are off. If you feel unhappy with this, keep the tips of your toes on the ground instead. With regular practice, your balance will improve.

BENEFITS

• In addition to the benefits for your bones, balance and self-confidence, Golden Pheasant also gently stimulates the energies of the Fire-element, promoting circulation, and physical and emotional warmth.

BEGIN BY slowly lowering your right arm and leg.

1 Your right foot goes flat on the ground as you lower your right arm to your side. Make sure your right foot settles alongside the left, about shoulder width from it and pointing outwards at an angle. Your right hand is relaxed, the palm facing downwards slightly.

2 Slowly raise your left knee to a comfortable height, along with your left arm. Again, your elbow finishes above your knee, and your forearm, elbow, knee and shin are in one vertical plane, not sticking out to one side or the other.

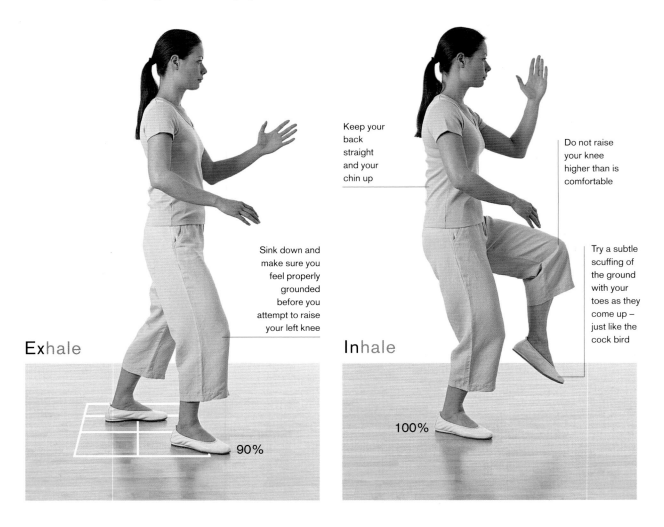

Keep your back straight and your chin up

Sink down and make sure you feel properly grounded before you attempt to raise your left knee

Exhale

90%

Do not raise your knee higher than is comfortable

Try a subtle scuffing of the ground with your toes as they come up – just like the cock bird

Inhale

100%

Pat the Horse, right side

Although the horse is one of the most powerful of animals, its movements in nature are often exceptionally graceful and fluent. Here, your arms emulate the movements of the horse's forelimbs when raised. It presents quite a challenge to your co-ordination, but feels very satisfying once mastered.

BENEFITS

• Mastering the slow, gradual descent from the Golden Pheasant into this movement is extremely effective in developing your balance and co-ordination.

• It also improves dexterity by encouraging you to use both upper and lower limbs simultaneously.

BEGIN BY relaxing your left arm and lowering your left foot towards the ground.

1 With your left foot contacting the ground, just slightly to the rear of the right, allow your weight to settle and drift back into your left side. The photograph shows the moment just before the weight moves into your left side.

2 Now continue to sweep up, forwards and across with your right palm, to rest (figuratively!) on the flank of a horse or pony. Your left palm, already turning upwards, settles at about waist level, as if holding an apple for the horse to eat. This whole movement should be smooth and rolling, so that your right forearm 'slides' over the left palm as it rises.

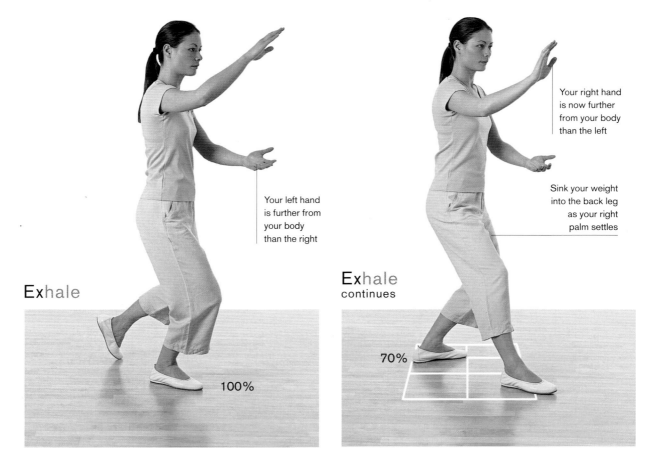

Your left hand is further from your body than the right

Your right hand is now further from your body than the left

Sink your weight into the back leg as your right palm settles

Exhale

100%

Exhale
continues

70%

Separate Hands and Kick with Right Toes

We now come to the first of a series of kicks. As with the punches you learned earlier, these movements remind us of tai chi's martial origins. However, do not get carried away with the idea of striking out at some imaginary foe. Aggression inevitably brings tension with it – and that is your real enemy. Stay calm.

BEGIN BY turning in your right heel slightly, as shown in the photograph to the right.

1 Drop both arms to a position level with your stomach. Your hands cross, left wrist over right and central. Both palms are facing inwards at this stage.

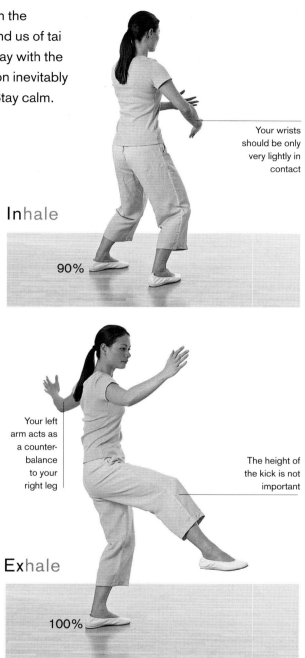

Your wrists should be only very lightly in contact

Inhale

90%

Prepare to draw up your knee by placing your weight in your left side

Inhale
continues

90%

Your left arm acts as a counter-balance to your right leg

The height of the kick is not important

Exhale

100%

2 Raise your arms, still crossed, to about chin height. At this stage, your wrists are about to roll so that your palms finish facing outwards. You are about to lift your right knee as well, so that your right foot leaves the ground. Make sure you feel properly balanced in your left foot first.

3 Separate out your hands, so that they describe a large arc in the air – the right hand going forwards, the left hand sliding back behind. Then straighten your right leg to complete the appearance of the kick, leading with the toes of your right foot. Allow your right hip to 'open' gently so that the leg rotates outwards slightly too, right of centre.

Pat the Horse, left side

You now repeat the movement on page 98, but this time as you pat the horse you will be leading with your left hand. After the kick, you take your next in-breath with your knee still raised. A tendency to lunge forward or topple after the kick exposes a weakness in your 'root', which can be corrected in this way.

BENEFITS

• Like its counterpart on page 98, this movement cultivates balance, co-ordination and resolve.

• It is particularly calming after the kicks, providing an opportunity to re-establish your root.

BEGIN BY allowing your shin to drop after the kick, but keeping your foot raised for a moment so that you can check your balance.

1 Place your right foot down carefully, heel first, slightly ahead of your left foot and on a diagonal. Your hands are drawn back towards the centre of your body, with the palms facing each other and the left palm a little higher than the right.

Take care to keep your shoulders level

Your right palm faces upwards, as if holding an apple for the horse to eat

Exhale

70%

Place the right foot down slowly, under control

Inhale

90%

2 Allow most of your weight to transfer forward into your right side, while your left hand glides and extends upwards to finish in an outward-facing position, left of centre at about chin height, as if resting on the horse's flank. Meanwhile, your right palm has fallen to around waist height, palm up. Allow your arms to move in graceful curves as you go.

Separate Hands and Kick with Left Toes

You now repeat the toe kick from page 99, but on the other side. As before, do not get carried away with the idea of kicking. Here you will be using the movement as an opportunity to gently stretch the top area of the leg and foot. It is also a further opportunity to test and to cultivate your sense of balance.

BENEFITS

• Like its counterpart on page 99, and indeed all other kicks in tai chi, this movement helps to develop your balance and self-confidence.

BEGIN BY stepping forward with your left foot so that it comes alongside your right.

1 Pivot on your left heel to go slightly pigeon-toed, while simultaneously shaping your hands and wrists into a cross-hands formation. Your right wrist rests on the left, with the palms facing inwards at about waist height. Next, roll your wrists outwards and upwards, just like you did on page 99. Your wrists are still crossed but your palms face outwards, ready for the next stage.

The 'kick' is performed very slowly, with your focus on the gentle stretch

Your right wrist rests on the left, now with the palms facing outwards below your chin

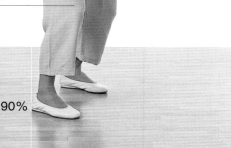

Exhale

100%

Your weight is settling into your right side, ready to raise your left knee

Inhale

90%

2 Raise your left knee, so that your lower leg hangs vertically above the ground. This preparation allows you to balance correctly before the kick. Next, separate your hands in another large, arc-like movement and then slowly raise your lower leg to create the appearance of a kick, leading with the toes of your left foot. Allow your left hip to 'open' gently so that the leg rotates outwards slightly too, left of centre.

Turn and Kick with the Sole

The next movement involves turning 180 degrees on your right heel, which can be done in a rather spectacular fashion without actually placing the left foot down at all. Here, however, you will be using a simplified version that takes in a little help from the left toes, in order to support some of your weight during the turn.

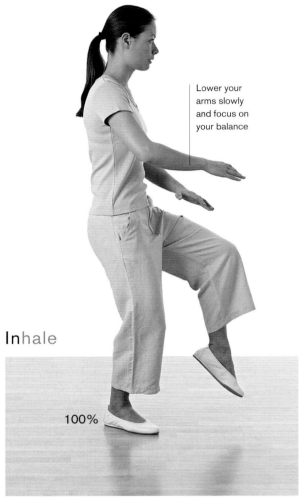

Lower your arms slowly and focus on your balance

Inhale

100%

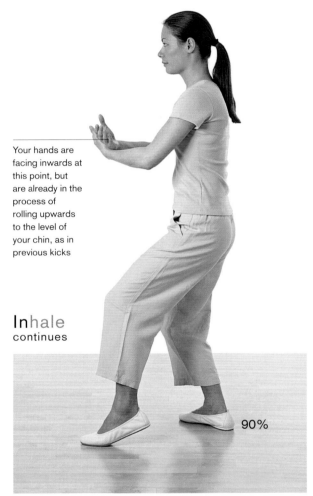

Your hands are facing inwards at this point, but are already in the process of rolling upwards to the level of your chin, as in previous kicks

Inhale continues

90%

BEGIN BY dropping your shin slowly and lowering your arms.

1 Start to breathe in and allow your left arm to drop slowly, almost vertical, across your centre, your right arm finishing a little higher outside your right hip. Your wrists are about to cross in just a moment. Meanwhile, your knee remains up, with your left foot still off the ground.

2 Pivoting on your right heel, open out your left hip and turn your waist counter-clockwise – just far enough to place the ball of your left foot on to the ground behind. Then transfer your weight into this foot, so that you can pivot further on your right heel to complete the rest of the 180-degree turn. As you go, your wrists cross right over left at stomach height, just before the weight begins to return to your right side.

BENEFITS

• The heel kick stimulates the hamstring and Achilles tendon in the back of the leg.

• It also affects the acu-channels relating to Kidney and Bladder energies, regulating fluids, cleansing the body of toxins and, it is believed, helping to establish a strong and decisive will.

• This movement can help you overcome anxiety and build self-confidence through increasing challenges to your balance.

Raise your left knee as your wrists roll upwards, then separate your hands in a graceful arc (which should be familiar to you by now), your left arm going forward and your right arm sliding back behind. Then project your left foot outwards to complete the appearance of the kick, although this time it is the sole of the foot rather than the toes that are exposed.

Your right arm goes behind to counter-balance your left leg

Remember that the 'kick' is done slowly – height is not important

Exhale

100%

Brush Left Knee and Push

The next few moves are ones you already know and so present an opportunity to add a whole lot more to your form in a short space of time. This movement repeats the exercise on pages 57 and 59, but this time you will be facing in the opposite direction and you are stepping down from a stance in which your weight is all in one leg.

BENEFITS

• This exercise will further increase your sense of balance and fluency of movement.

• It also continues to build strength in the muscles, tendons and bones of your legs and hips.

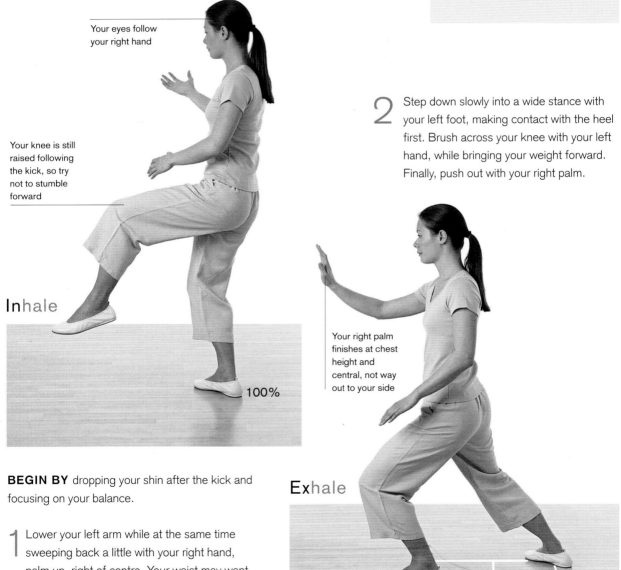

Your eyes follow your right hand

Your knee is still raised following the kick, so try not to stumble forward

Inhale

100%

2 Step down slowly into a wide stance with your left foot, making contact with the heel first. Brush across your knee with your left hand, while bringing your weight forward. Finally, push out with your right palm.

Your right palm finishes at chest height and central, not way out to your side

Exhale

70%

BEGIN BY dropping your shin after the kick and focusing on your balance.

1 Lower your left arm while at the same time sweeping back a little with your right hand, palm up, right of centre. Your waist may want to rotate a little clockwise as you circle slightly behind with your right palm.

Brush Right Knee and Push

This is the first time you have encountered this movement on the right side, and you will notice straight away the difference in your fluency compared to the left-sided version, which you have already practised a lot by this stage. This disparity shows what a difference regular practice can make.

BEGIN BY establishing the Yin phase of the movement (see page 17) by sitting back and turning out the toes of your left foot.

BENEFITS

• This sequence is very helpful in learning to how to focus and use your energies more economically, changing as needed from one limb to the other, one hand to the other.

• It also develops strength and muscle tone in the thighs.

1 Lower your right arm to your centre while circling your left palm back behind your shoulder, palm up. Allow your waist to rotate a little counter-clockwise to accommodate this movement, and at the same time prepare to raise your right foot from the ground by bringing your weight into your left side.

2 Step forward with your right foot, heel first, and bend your knee to bring your weight forward. As you step, brush your right knee with your right palm, the hand travelling from left to right in a sweeping motion. Then push out with your left palm, at chest height and only slightly right of centre.

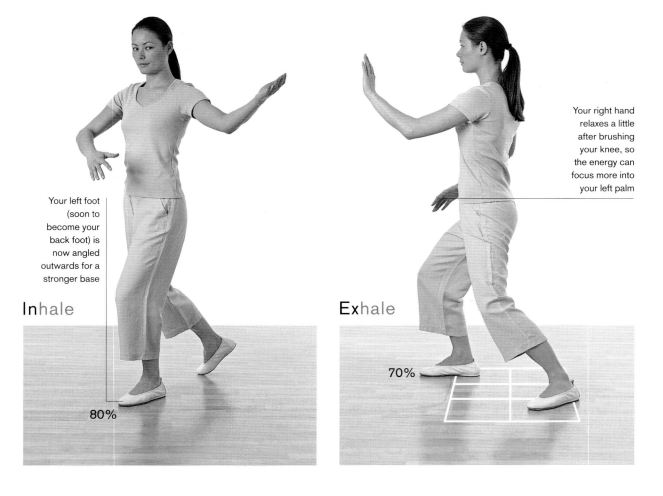

Your left foot (soon to become your back foot) is now angled outwards for a stronger base

Inhale

80%

Your right hand relaxes a little after brushing your knee, so the energy can focus more into your left palm

Exhale

70%

Brush Left Knee and Punch Low

Similar to Brush Left Knee and Push, the difference here is that instead of pushing out with your right palm, you form a fist in your right hand and project this downwards at the conclusion of the step. The footwork follows the same pattern, turning out what is to become the back foot first, then stepping forward.

BEGIN BY establishing the Yin phase of the movement (see page 17) by sitting back and turning out the toes of your right foot.

1 Bring your weight into your right side and raise your left foot, ready to step forward into a wide stance. Your waist may want to turn just a little clockwise as you form a fist with your right hand. The knuckles are facing upwards this time, so it is different to the prelude to the punch on page 61. Meanwhile, your left hand has drifted in towards your centre.

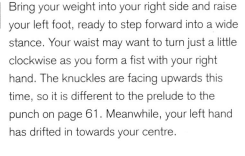

This front view shows that the hand is loose and relaxed, knuckles facing upwards

Make sure your back does not bend as you punch low.

Exhale

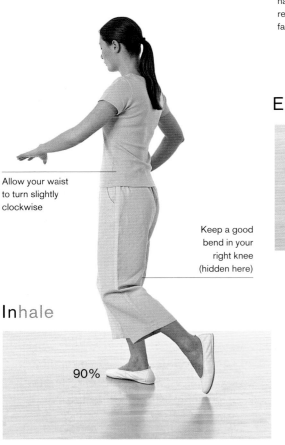

Allow your waist to turn slightly clockwise

Keep a good bend in your right knee (hidden here)

Inhale

90%

70%

2 Step forward into a wide stance and bend your left knee as the weight goes forward. As you go, your left palm brushes over your left thigh in the usual way. Finally, extend your right hand in the form of a slow punch, spiralling downwards and central to about knee height, your fist rotating as it goes to finish thumb-side up. If you feel your back bending as you punch, simply straighten up and 'punch' at a higher level. Alternatively, let your body sink down, as if between your knees.

Grasp the Bird's Tail

Still using the same technique of stepping forward, you now encounter a further repetition of the Chorus, first seen on pages 47 to 53 and with which you should be familiar by now. The whole routine follows on easily from the forward-stepping sequence established in the previous few movements.

BEGIN BY establishing the Yin phase of the movement (see page 17) by sitting back and turning out the toes of your left foot.

1 Bring the weight into your left side and raise your right foot, ready to step forward into another wide stance. Rotate your waist counter-clockwise and pick up a ball, left hand on top, right hand underneath. Keep your back upright as your waist turns.

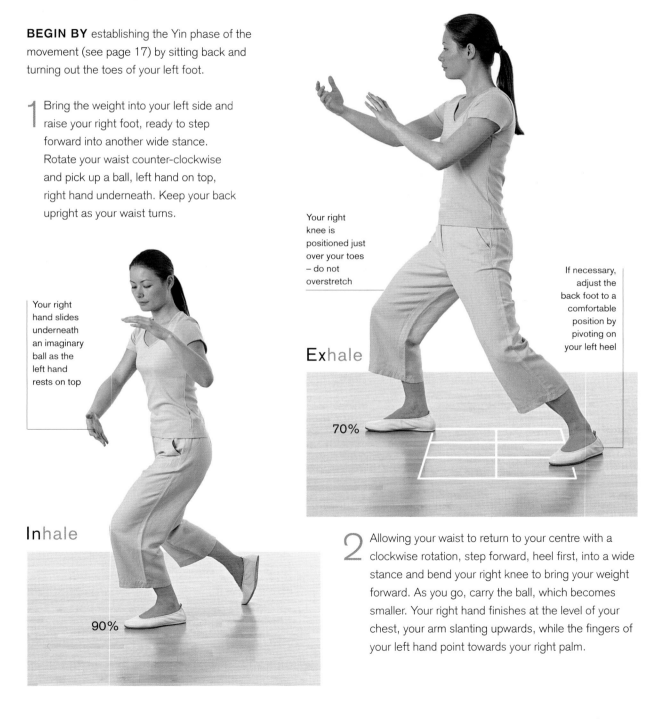

Your right hand slides underneath an imaginary ball as the left hand rests on top

Your right knee is positioned just over your toes – do not overstretch

If necessary, adjust the back foot to a comfortable position by pivoting on your left heel

Exhale

70%

Inhale

90%

2 Allowing your waist to return to your centre with a clockwise rotation, step forward, heel first, into a wide stance and bend your right knee to bring your weight forward. As you go, carry the ball, which becomes smaller. Your right hand finishes at the level of your chest, your arm slanting upwards, while the fingers of your left hand point towards your right palm.

The Chorus

The tai chi sequence continues with a repetition of movements learned on pages 48–53. You should be comfortable with these, so they are illustrated on a smaller scale. The order is the same: Grasp the Bird's Tail (see page 107) is followed by Rollback and Press, then Separate Hands and Push, and finally the Single Whip.

Your spine should remain upright throughout. Try to resist the temptation to speed up with these movements simply because you are already familiar with them. It is this constant repetition of well-rehearsed movements, without conscious thought, that enables you to 'let go' and approach the Chinese philosophers' concept of Wu Wei (no mind). This is also getting nearer to experiencing that special 'moving meditation' state of mind. So, keep the rhythm of your movements slow, and the breath that guides them constant from start to finish.

Rollback and Press

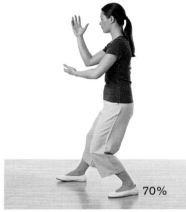

1 Inhale

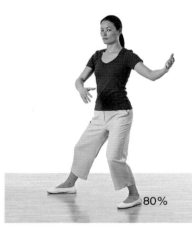

2 Inhale continues

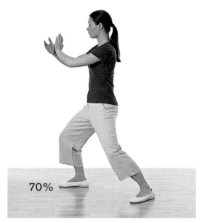

3 Exhale

Separate Hands and Push

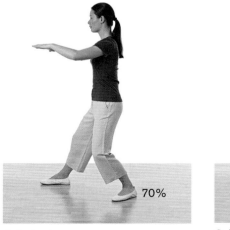

1 Inhale

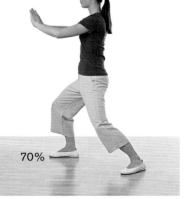

2 Exhale

Single Whip

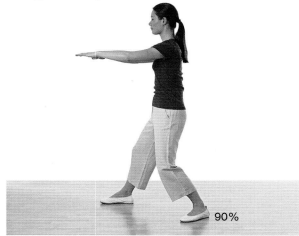

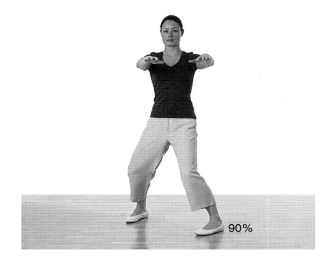

1 Inhale

2 Exhale

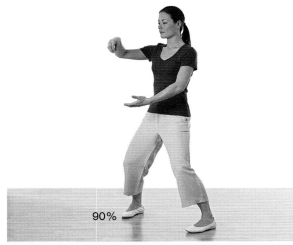

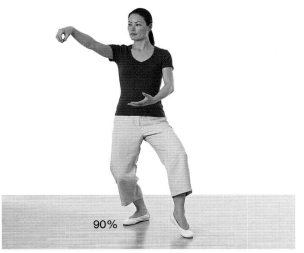

3 Inhale

4 Exhale

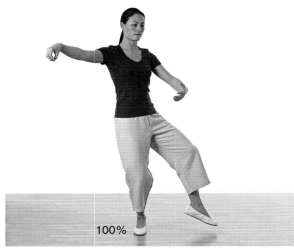

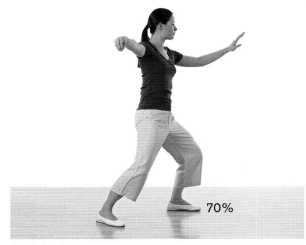

5 Inhale

6 Exhale

Four Corners – first

The Four Corners sequence is almost like a small tai chi form in itself. It consists of four separate movements, each one lasting for two whole breaths, and starting and finishing on a diagonal – facing a 'corner'. They are beautiful to watch, and are some of the most enjoyable and satisfying of all the movements to do.

BEGIN BY letting go of the crane's beak and shifting your weight into your right side.

1 Pivot a little on your left heel to point your toes inwards. Your waist rotates clockwise as your right hand turns, so that the palm begins to face your body. Meanwhile, your left hand drops slowly down to your centre, palm up, following your waist as it turns.

2 Bring your weight into your left foot and raise your right foot, ready to step. Continue to rotate your waist clockwise and then place your right foot slowly flat onto the ground in the position shown. This allows you to restore your weight once again to your right side.

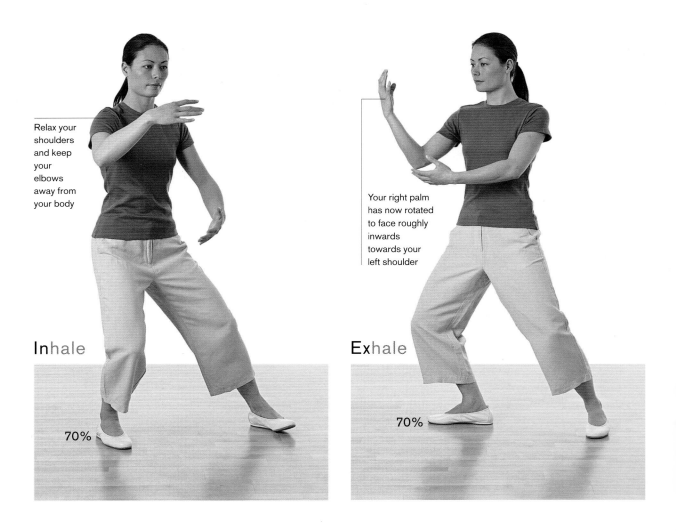

Relax your shoulders and keep your elbows away from your body

Inhale

70%

Your right palm has now rotated to face roughly inwards towards your left shoulder

Exhale

70%

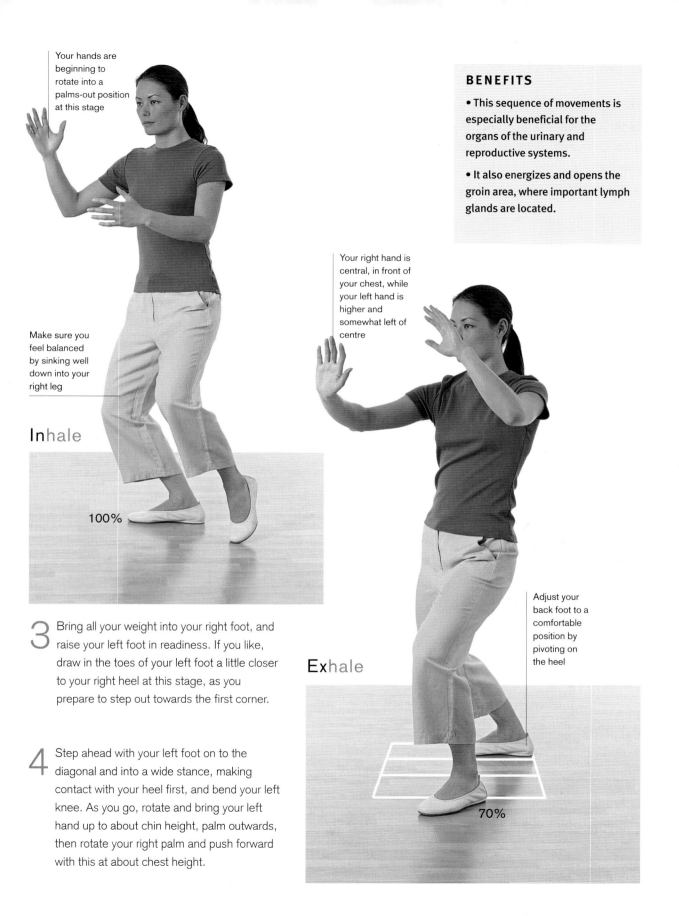

Your hands are beginning to rotate into a palms-out position at this stage

Make sure you feel balanced by sinking well down into your right leg

Inhale

100%

BENEFITS

• This sequence of movements is especially beneficial for the organs of the urinary and reproductive systems.

• It also energizes and opens the groin area, where important lymph glands are located.

Your right hand is central, in front of your chest, while your left hand is higher and somewhat left of centre

Exhale

Adjust your back foot to a comfortable position by pivoting on the heel

70%

3 Bring all your weight into your right foot, and raise your left foot in readiness. If you like, draw in the toes of your left foot a little closer to your right heel at this stage, as you prepare to step out towards the first corner.

4 Step ahead with your left foot on to the diagonal and into a wide stance, making contact with your heel first, and bend your left knee. As you go, rotate and bring your left hand up to about chin height, palm outwards, then rotate your right palm and push forward with this at about chest height.

Four Corners – second

The second corner calls for some challenging footwork, to enable
you to turn through a full 270 degrees (three-quarters of a circle).
If you think of the first corner as having finished facing, say,
south-west on the compass, this one will finish facing south-east.
You turn clockwise – the long route – to reach it.

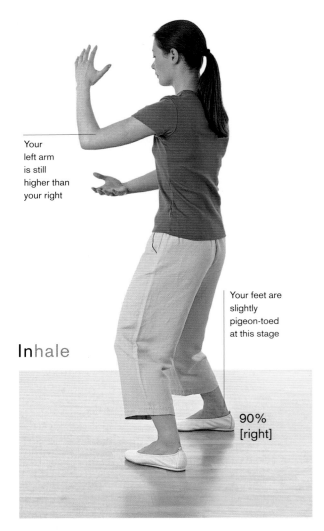

Your
left arm
is still
higher than
your right

Your feet are
slightly
pigeon-toed
at this stage

Inhale

90%
[right]

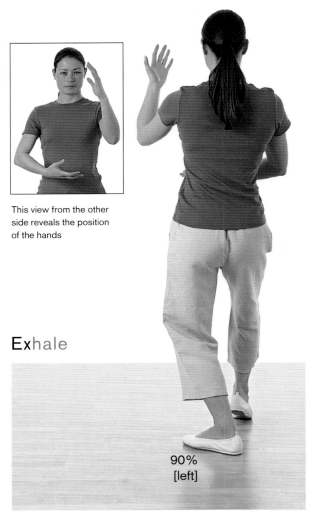

This view from the other
side reveals the position
of the hands

Exhale

90%
[left]

BEGIN BY transferring your weight into the back leg.
Sit back and relax.

1 Turn your waist clockwise and pivot a little on your left
heel to point your toes inwards. Rotate your palms
slowly inwards again and draw your arms back a little
closer to your body. Your right hand drops slowly down
to your centre, close to your left elbow, palm up.

2 Bring your weight into your left foot, sinking into it,
and continue to rotate your waist clockwise by raising
your right heel and pivoting on your toes. Your left
palm has now rotated to face roughly towards your
right shoulder.

3 Bring all your weight into your left foot and raise your right foot completely from the ground. Keep turning your waist clockwise, way around to your right-hand side, as you prepare to step out towards the second corner. Let the inhalation open your shoulders for you, and keep your back straight.

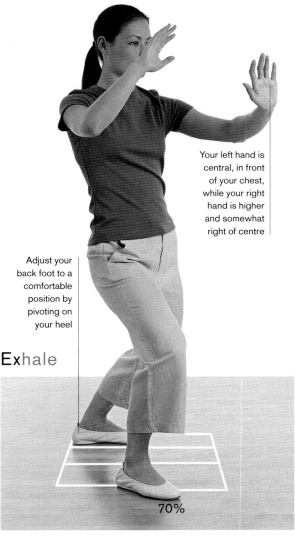

Your hands are beginning to rotate into a palms-out position at this stage

Make sure you feel balanced by sinking well down into your left leg

Inhale

100% [left]

Your left hand is central, in front of your chest, while your right hand is higher and somewhat right of centre

Adjust your back foot to a comfortable position by pivoting on your heel

Exhale

70%

4 Step around with your right foot on to the diagonal into a wide stance, making contact with your heel first, and bend your right knee. As you go, rotate and bring your right hand up to about chin height, palm outwards, then rotate your left palm and push forward with this at about chest height.

Four Corners – third

The third corner is more straightforward. You just step over directly to it. Referring to compass directions again, if the previous corner finished facing south-east, this one will be to the north-east. Incidentally, there is a useful rule: as you come to the end of each corner, the higher arm is always on the side with the leading leg.

BEGIN BY transferring your weight into your back leg. Sit back and relax.

1 Your right hand turns so that the palm begins to face your body. Meanwhile, your left hand drops lower, down to your centre and close to your right elbow, palm up, following your waist as it turns. Begin to raise your right foot, ready to step, and let your waist turn just a little counter-clockwise.

2 With all your weight in your left side, step forwards and slightly across to place your right foot down flat on the ground in front of your left foot.

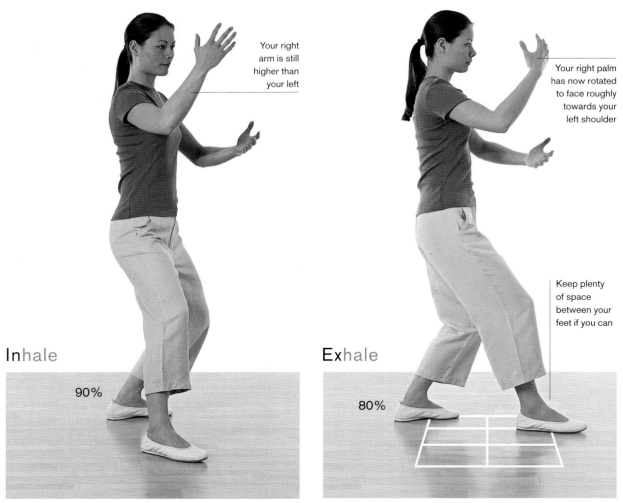

Your right arm is still higher than your left

Your right palm has now rotated to face roughly towards your left shoulder

Keep plenty of space between your feet if you can

Inhale

90%

Exhale

80%

3 Prepare to step out towards the diagonal by raising your left foot. Your arms start to open up again now, ready for the final step. Think of your left palm running up the outside of your right forearm, though at a distance, as your palms begin to rotate outwards.

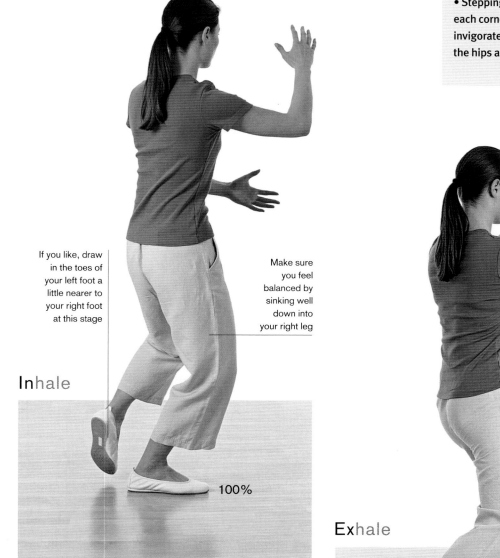

Your right hand is central, in front of your chest, while your left hand is higher and somewhat left of centre

If you like, draw in the toes of your left foot a little nearer to your right foot at this stage

Make sure you feel balanced by sinking well down into your right leg

Inhale

100%

Exhale

70%

4 Step out with your left foot on to the diagonal into a wide stance, making contact with your heel first, and bend your left knee. As you go, rotate and bring up your left palm to about chin height, facing outwards, then rotate your right palm and push forward with this at about chest height.

Four Corners – fourth

The fourth and final corner takes the long route around once more – this time heading for the north-west corner according to your imaginary compass. So, make use of that special combination of turning on heels and toes, and keep rotating your waist clockwise to help you on your way.

BEGIN BY transferring your weight into your rear leg. Sit back and relax.

1 Turn your waist clockwise and pivot a little on your left heel to point the toes inwards. Rotate your palms slowly inwards again and draw your arms back a little closer to your body. Your right hand drops slowly down to your centre, close to your left elbow, palm up.

2 Bring your weight into your left foot and continue to rotate your waist clockwise by raising your right heel and pivoting on your toes. Your left palm has now rotated to face roughly towards your right shoulder.

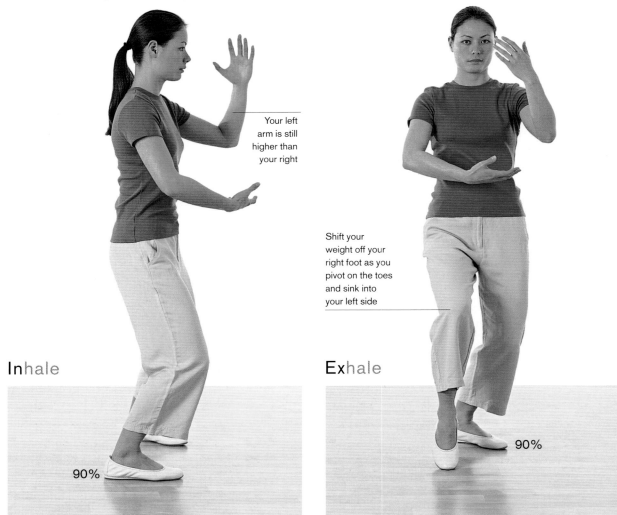

Your left arm is still higher than your right

Shift your weight off your right foot as you pivot on the toes and sink into your left side

Inhale

Exhale

90%

90%

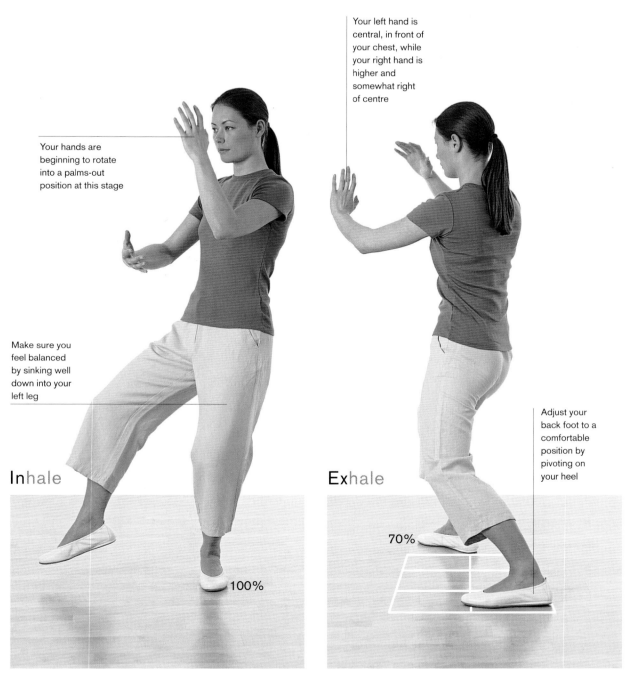

Your hands are beginning to rotate into a palms-out position at this stage

Your left hand is central, in front of your chest, while your right hand is higher and somewhat right of centre

Make sure you feel balanced by sinking well down into your left leg

Adjust your back foot to a comfortable position by pivoting on your heel

Inhale

Exhale

100%

70%

3 Bring all your weight into your left foot and raise your right foot completely off the ground. Keep turning your waist clockwise, way around to your right-hand side, as you prepare to step out towards the fourth corner. Let the inhalation open your shoulders for you, and keep your back straight.

4 Open your hip and step around with your right foot on to the diagonal and into a wide stance, making contact with your heel first, and bend your right knee. As you go, rotate and bring up your right palm to about chin height, facing outwards, then rotate your left palm and push forward with this at about chest height.

Ward Off

From your final Corner, all you need to do now is repeat a movement already learned, way back on page 46. The only difference here is that you are coming to it from a diagonal, so your feet have to work that little bit harder.

way back on page 46

BEGIN BY relaxing your arms, transferring your weight back into your left foot and pivoting inwards slightly on your right heel.

1 Lower your left arm slowly down to your centre as you rotate your waist counter-clockwise. Your right palm begins to rotate inwards. Then return your weight into your right side, ready to raise your left foot to step forward.

BENEFITS

• Like all wide stances, this movement establishes a solid foundation for your posture.

• It also improves your balance and self-confidence, and gives you a feel for the 'grounding' quality of tai chi – beneficial in dancing, sports and even in helping to prevent the elderly from falling.

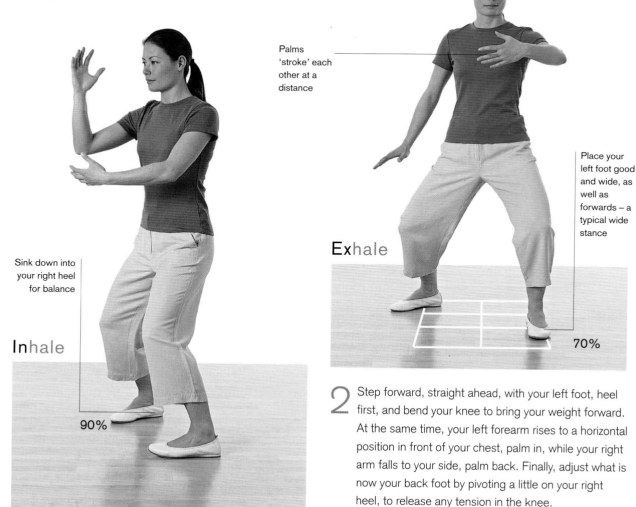

Palms 'stroke' each other at a distance

Sink down into your right heel for balance

Inhale

90%

Exhale

Place your left foot good and wide, as well as forwards – a typical wide stance

70%

2 Step forward, straight ahead, with your left foot, heel first, and bend your knee to bring your weight forward. At the same time, your left forearm rises to a horizontal position in front of your chest, palm in, while your right arm falls to your side, palm back. Finally, adjust what is now your back foot by pivoting a little on your right heel, to release any tension in the knee.

Chorus

After Ward Off you continue with one final Chorus, beginning with Grasp the Bird's Tail. With this you can add yet another huge chunk to the overall sequence. You should know all these movements well by now, so we illustrate them here once more on a smaller scale. If you are in any doubt, refer to pages 47–53.

One of the advantages in having a repeated sequence like the Chorus (it occurs four times in all) is that it provides a kind of land-mark along the way, a place of reference – invaluable when you are trying to memorize the whole form.

These movements have always been thought of as especially valuable – and this is still true, whether you are an enthusiast of tai chi's martial aspects or whether, like us, you are simply interested in promoting better health.

Grasp the Bird's Tail

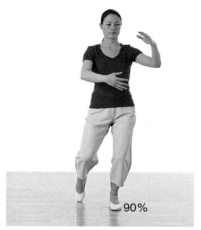

1 Inhale

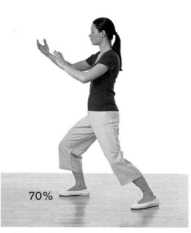

2 Exhale

Rollback and Press

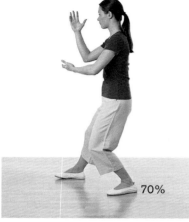

1 Inhale

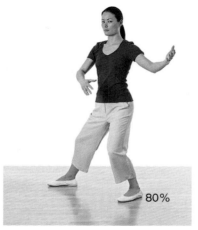

2 Inhale continues

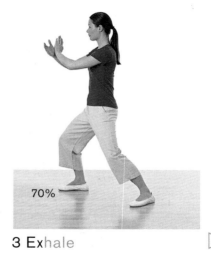

3 Exhale

Separate Hands and Push

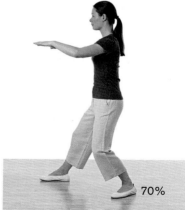

1 Inhale

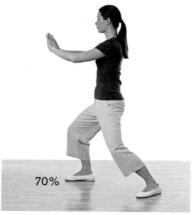

2 Exhale

Single Whip

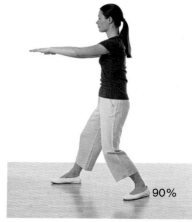

1 Inhale

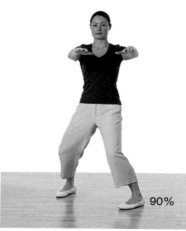

2 Exhale

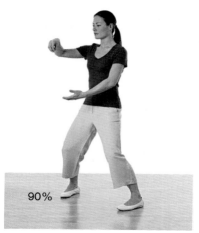

3 Inhale

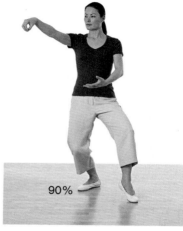

4 Exhale

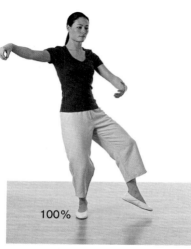

5 Inhale

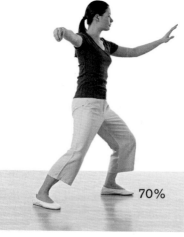

6 Exhale

Snake Creeps Down

From the final Chorus, the tai chi sequence continues with a repetition of another movement you have already learned. This is Snake Creeps Down – sometimes also called the Squatting Single Whip. This movement is shown again in full.

BENEFITS

• This movement vigorously exercises the joints of the hips, knees and ankles.

• It gently tones the muscles of the upper thigh and buttocks.

BEGIN BY relaxing your left hand and bringing most of your weight temporarily forward into your left foot.

1 Lengthen your stance by sliding back with your right foot. Then return your weight to your right foot, rotate your waist clockwise and bend your right knee, to 'squat' down on the back leg. Meanwhile, your left palm traces back to a position roughly facing your chest.

Your back knee is positioned directly over your foot for stability

Inhale

90%

2 Pivot a little on your left heel if you can, to point your toes inwards, as you continue to sink down and squat on your right knee. Your waist continues to rotate clockwise, and your left hand has progressed down in a graceful arc to a position close to your right leg.

Keep your right arm extended but not tense

Unless you are able, do not feel that you have to squat down too far

Inhale continues

90%

3 Your left hand now continues its journey by thrusting forward, close to the ground, as you realign your front foot by pointing the toes straight ahead again. If you were to trace its path through the air, you would find that the left hand roughly describes a large clockwise circle back, down and forward during this movement.

Exhale

Your left foot straightens once more

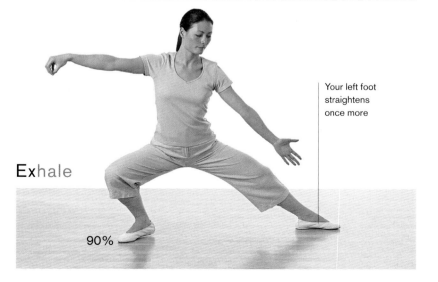

90%

Step Forward to Seven Stars

Some say that the 'seven stars' here are the seven most visible stars of the Great Bear, or Plough. If you look at this stance in profile, it does resemble the shape of the constellation we call Ursa Major. This is the first of several exciting movements that feature in the final part of the form.

BENEFITS

• This dynamic movement strengthens the legs and provides helpful rotations for the wrist and elbow joints.

• In common with many tai chi movements, the strong, purposeful aspect of the hands also provides a further means of developing better concentration and mental focus.

BEGIN BY shifting your weight forward and pivoting inwards once more on your right heel.

1 Turn out your left foot to form a comfortable base for what comes next, then bring yourself out of the squat by drawing your body forward and up. You can now start to think of forming a cross-wrists formation with your hands that will be left wrist over right.

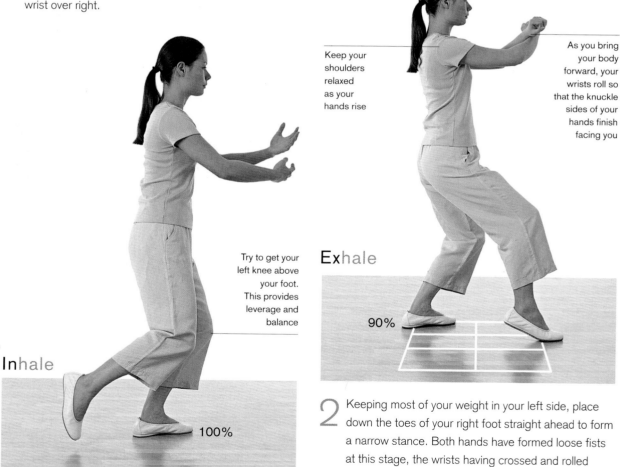

Keep your shoulders relaxed as your hands rise

As you bring your body forward, your wrists roll so that the knuckle sides of your hands finish facing you

Try to get your left knee above your foot. This provides leverage and balance

Exhale

90%

Inhale

100%

2 Keeping most of your weight in your left side, place down the toes of your right foot straight ahead to form a narrow stance. Both hands have formed loose fists at this stage, the wrists having crossed and rolled upwards from waist height to about chin height. You should be looking out over your crossed wrists as if towards a distant horizon.

Step Back to Ride the Tiger

By now you may have noticed that the tiger appears quite often in the naming of tai chi movements. A creature of strength and vital energy, the tiger is also the mightiest of opponents – perhaps signifying that our greatest strength and our greatest adversary both lie within ourselves.

BEGIN BY uncrossing your wrists and lowering your hands just a little.

1 With your weight still in your left side, step back with your right foot, making contact with your toes first. Then bring your weight into your right foot and raise your left heel to form a narrow toe stance, this time on the left. Meanwhile, your hands separate out, the left dropping to just left of centre and the right spiralling out and up again to about head height.

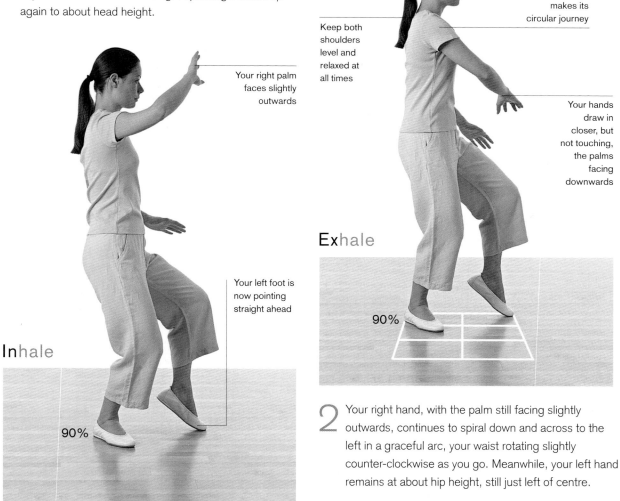

Your right palm faces slightly outwards

Keep both shoulders level and relaxed at all times

Do not tense your right shoulder as your right hand makes its circular journey

Your hands draw in closer, but not touching, the palms facing downwards

Your left foot is now pointing straight ahead

Inhale

90%

Exhale

90%

2 Your right hand, with the palm still facing slightly outwards, continues to spiral down and across to the left in a graceful arc, your waist rotating slightly counter-clockwise as you go. Meanwhile, your left hand remains at about hip height, still just left of centre.

Sweep the Lotus and Crescent Kick

The next movement involves a full 360-degree turn, using a combination of pivoting on heels and toes. The oriental lotus flower is an aquatic plant and here you are going to sweep the flower from the surface of the pool. The movement finishes with a 'kick' and is one of the most challenging in the entire tai chi form.

BEGIN BY lifting your left foot from the ground and straightening your leg, ready to 'sweep'.

1 Making use of the momentum of your arms and left leg, sweep your body around in a clockwise direction, turning on the ball of your right foot and leading with the outer edge of your left foot.

2 Touch down behind with your left foot, making contact with the heel first. You are now, for a moment, facing the opposite direction from which you began the movement. Although your weight is all in your right side during the turn, in the photograph it is just beginning to shift into the left foot as this makes contact with the ground.

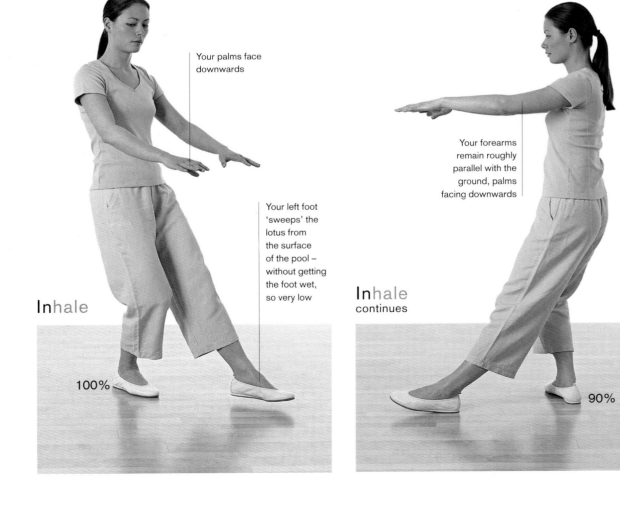

Your palms face downwards

Your left foot 'sweeps' the lotus from the surface of the pool – without getting the foot wet, so very low

Inhale

100%

Your forearms remain roughly parallel with the ground, palms facing downwards

Inhale continues

90%

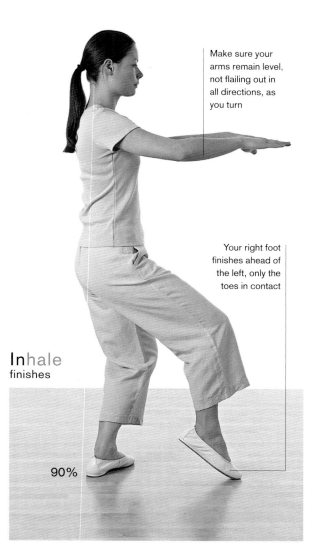

Make sure your arms remain level, not flailing out in all directions, as you turn

Your right foot finishes ahead of the left, only the toes in contact

Inhale
finishes

90%

BENEFITS

• This movement builds flexibility in your spine, knees and hips.

• Extremely challenging, it will increase your self-confidence and balance.

• It also stimulates the rear aspect of the leg and therefore the Kidney and Bladder energies.

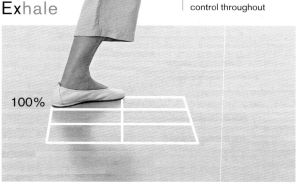

As your leg sweeps right, your arms may move slightly in the other direction, palms still facing downwards and wrists relaxed

The height of the kick is not important – concentrate instead on maintaining a sense of balance and control throughout

Exhale

100%

3 Continue the turn, all the way around to the direction in which you were facing at the start, by pivoting on the ball of your right foot and the heel of your left. Your forearms, meanwhile, remain roughly horizontal, palms facing down. All this has to be done fairly quickly, especially when you are learning, but it is surprising how graceful and accomplished you will become with continued practice.

4 With your forearms just a little right of centre, raise your right knee and then, as your shin also comes up to create the straightened aspect to the leg, sweep your right foot outwards in an arc (crescent shape). If your foot were to be making contact with anything, therefore, it would be the outer edge that would do so.

Crescent Kick conclusion

Following any kick, you need to take an in-breath before setting the foot down again. This ensures that you are still in control of the process. Simply toppling forward into the next movement is not good enough. The in-breath at the start of this movement gives you time to pause, and helps to settle the energies.

BEGIN BY dropping your shin and turning your waist slightly clockwise to align your body with your right thigh.

1 With your knee still raised, allow your arms to settle above your right thigh, palms still facing downwards. Take your time, regaining full composure after the spectacular work you have just completed.

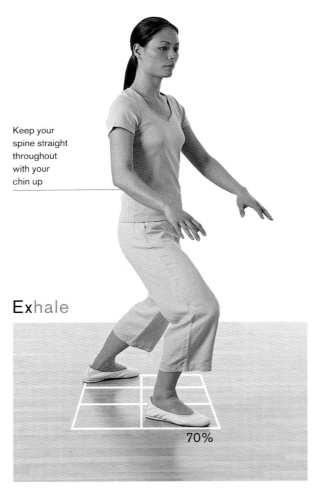

Keep your spine straight throughout with your chin up

Exhale

70%

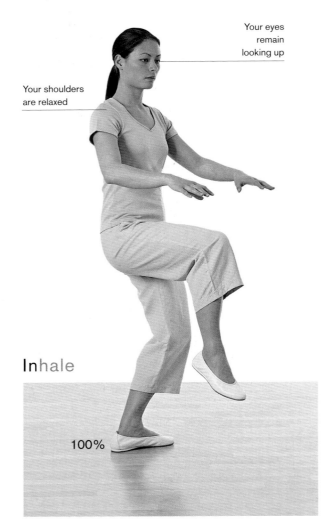

Your eyes remain looking up

Your shoulders are relaxed

Inhale

100%

2 Set your foot down slowly, making contact with the heel first, the toes pointing outwards. Bend your right knee, sink down and bring your weight forward into your right side. Allow your hands to drift across your thigh and drop down just a little at the end. Relax.

Bend the Bow and Shoot the Tiger

In this movement your hands form very loose fists, or appear to be curled around a bow or staff. If you are just starting to practise tai chi, the action of the right arm can cause your right shoulder to rise up and become tense. It is important to monitor your actions closely and keep your shoulders level at all times.

BENEFITS

• This interesting movement develops your sense of balance and enhances the sense of an energetic connection between your hands.

• It also increases flexibility in the joints of your shoulders, elbows and wrists.

BEGIN BY closing your hands very loosely around an imaginary bow or staff, your forearms still horizontal and the knuckle side of your hands still uppermost.

1 Glide your right hand upwards and inwards in a graceful curve to about head height. As your hand rises, it rotates so that the knuckles turn inwards. This means that your arm has a gentle twist or spiral shape along its length. Keep the relationship between your hands intact – that is, still holding that imaginary staff or bow between them.

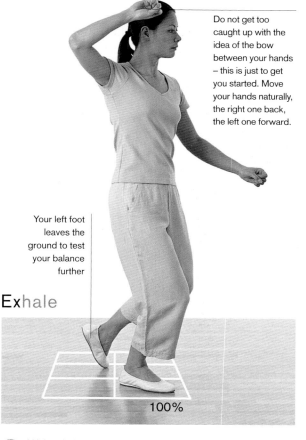

Do not get too caught up with the idea of the bow between your hands – this is just to get you started. Move your hands naturally, the right one back, the left one forward.

Your left foot leaves the ground to test your balance further

Exhale

100%

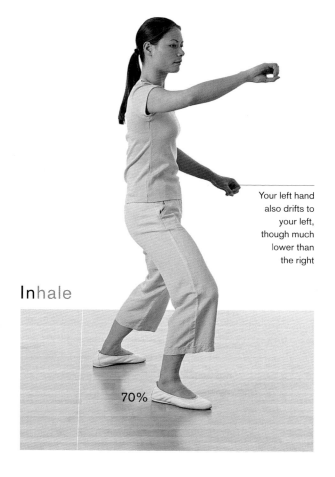

Your left hand also drifts to your left, though much lower than the right

Inhale

70%

2 With a little clockwise rotation to your waist, 'bend the bow' – that is, draw your right hand back to a position close to the side of your head while projecting your left hand forward, left of centre. Finally, as your waist turns to accommodate the arm movements, bring your back foot off the ground and forward a little by bending your knee.

Step Forward, Parry and Punch

You have met this movement already on pages 60–61, towards the end of part 1 of the form. It appears here once more to initiate the closing sequence of part 2 and, therefore, of the whole form. The main difference here is that previously the sequence began with the left foot forward, whereas here you start with the right foot forward.

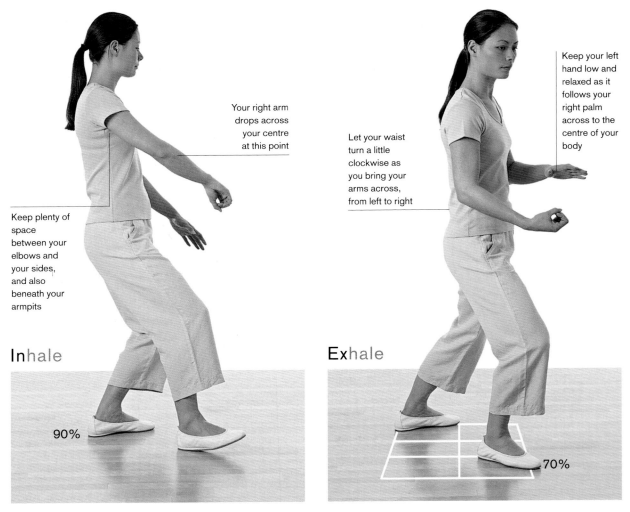

Your right arm drops across your centre at this point

Keep plenty of space between your elbows and your sides, and also beneath your armpits

Let your waist turn a little clockwise as you bring your arms across, from left to right

Keep your left hand low and relaxed as it follows your right palm across to the centre of your body

Inhale

90%

Exhale

70%

BEGIN BY placing your left foot down flat on the ground and allowing your weight to return to it.

1 Let go of the fist in your left hand, but retain the one in your right. Gently lower your arms, your left hand going down and around to your left side, your right hand finishing just left of centre. Begin to raise your right foot by lifting the toes.

2 Lift your right foot for a moment and then set it down again at more of an angle, still ahead of your left but with the toes pointing further out than before. This will provide a firm base for the next stage as you step forward. Simultaneously, 'throw' your right fist around to your right side, palm side uppermost, allowing your left hand to follow it. Finally, sink into your right leg and bend your knee.

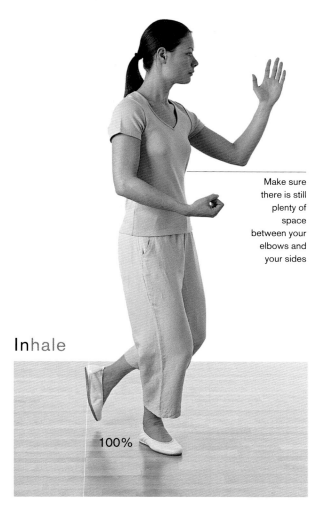

Make sure there is still plenty of space between your elbows and your sides

Inhale

100%

3 Prepare to step forward by bringing all your weight into your right side and drawing in the toes of your left foot just a little towards your right heel. Then lift your left forearm, ready for the parry, and draw back the fist in your right hand, knuckles still facing downwards, ready for the 'punch'.

Keep a little softness in your elbow, even at the end of the movement

Adjust your back heel to a comfortable position as your weight goes forward

Exhale

70%

4 Step ahead with your left foot and bend your knee. At the same time, sweep your left forearm away from your centre to the left and then project your right hand forward in the 'punch'. Do this by simply unbending your right elbow. Your right hand rotates in mid-flight to finish with the thumb-side uppermost.

Release Arm and Push

You now continue winding up the tai chi form with the same routine as used on pages 62–63. We show the sequence again here, this time with a different model so that you can see the subtle differences every individual brings to these movements. Observe how, in both cases, the movement is initiated by the rotation of the waist.

BEGIN BY relaxing your arms and turning your waist just a little counter-clockwise.

1 Draw your right hand, still in a fist, across to a position left of centre, with your forearm more or less horizontal. Then slide your left hand beneath your right forearm and beyond, the fingers pointing forwards and the palm facing downwards for the moment.

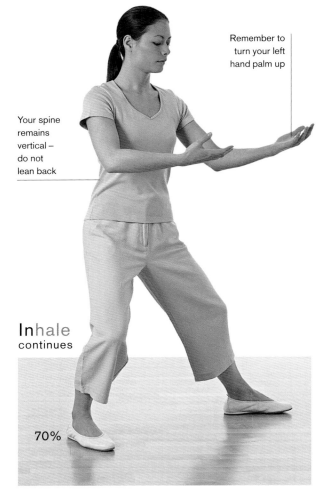

Remember to turn your left hand palm up

Your spine remains vertical – do not lean back

Inhale continues

70%

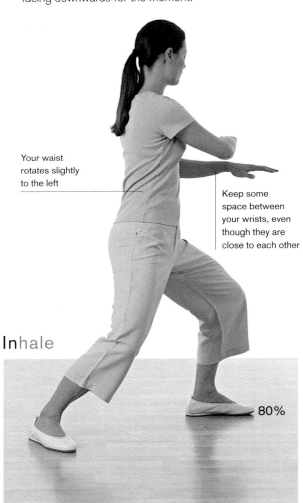

Your waist rotates slightly to the left

Keep some space between your wrists, even though they are close to each other

Inhale

80%

2 Now let go of the fist and rotate both wrists into a palms-up position. Shift your weight back and rotate your waist clockwise, while simultaneously drawing your right hand back across your left forearm. This appears to 'release' your right arm and set it free from the left, but the expansive character of the movement is actually achieved by the action of your waist and the shifting of your weight to the back leg.

BENEFITS

• Rotations of the wrist have their origin at the elbow, so this movement can retain the suppleness and strength of this joint and avoid problems like 'tennis elbow'.

• The intricacy of the movement will also improve your dexterity and confidence in your ability.

3 Prepare to push out by turning both palms to face forwards and rotating your centre to also face straight ahead. The push that concludes this movement is similar to the one that occurs in the Chorus, except that here your left foot is forward instead of the right. Simply return your weight to your front leg by bending the knee and make the push shape with your hands.

Do not thrust forward with your palms – just use the bend of your knee to create the 'push'

Keep the bottom tucked in, so maintaining a straight spine

Front knee just above the toes – no further!

Exhale

70%

Turn and Close part 2

The closing of part 2, and indeed of the whole form, is exactly the same as the closing of part 1, already encountered on pages 64–67. Try not to speed up or become too keen to reach the end. With tai chi you maintain the same even pace throughout, slowly, evenly, from start to finish.

BEGIN BY transferring a good percentage of your weight back into your right leg.

1 Relax your hands and pivot slowly on your left heel to help turn your waist clockwise, returning to face in your original opening direction. The aspect of your hands here is initially rather like somebody warming their hands at a fire, palms forward and facing slightly downwards, but as you turn they begin to lift a little and separate out from each other.

Your energy is focused more in your right hand at this stage

Your hands should be relaxed, gliding gently apart

Exhale

Inhale

90%

90%

2 Allow your hands to continue separating, forming an ever-widening arc that in a moment will become a full circle. Transfer your weight back into your left side and rotate your body clockwise 90 degrees, then raise your right heel and begin drawing back your right foot into a position parallel with your left.

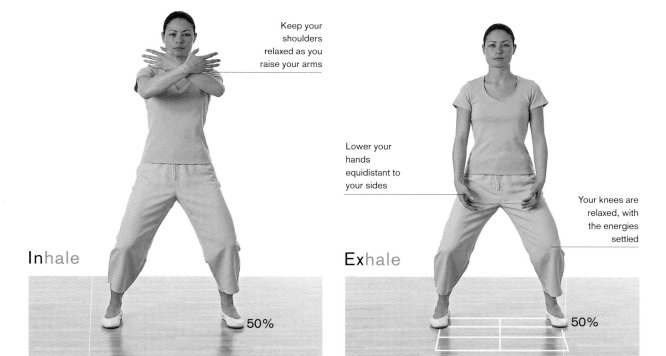

3 Your hands continue on their circular journey, down and then inwards once more to meet (without touching) in front of your lower abdomen. Return half your weight into your right side now, making for a rare 50/50 stance – though similar to those found at the start and end of part 1, of course. Your palms should be facing inwards at this stage, the fingers relaxed.

BENEFITS

• This final movement promotes relaxation and flexibility in the joints of the shoulders and the upper arms.

• It also stimulates areas of lymphatic tissue concentrated in the neck, chest and armpits.

• Finally, it allows you to take an important moment of rest following the rigours of the tai chi form.

As soon as your right foot is in position, let your weight return to it

Exhale
continues

50%

Keep your shoulders relaxed as you raise your arms

Inhale

50%

Lower your hands equidistant to your sides

Exhale

Your knees are relaxed, with the energies settled

50%

4 With the next in-breath, your hands begin to rise together with palms in, up through your centre until they cross, left wrist resting for a moment very lightly upon the right at about chin height. Your left forearm is therefore closer to you than the right as your wrists cross.

5 To finish, simply lower your arms gently down through your centre, allowing them to separate naturally as they fall to your sides. Sink down a little as you breath out, before completing your tai chi session. This can take the form of one or two extra breaths if you like, and also a moment's reflection on the sensations that remain after completing the tai chi journey.

A Summary of Movements

The photographs on the following pages show the whole form in miniature, in exactly the sequence you will be performing it. Once you have studied and assimilated the individual movements, use these summaries as a guide to help you go all the way through the sequence without pause. Remember that although tai chi has to be learned as separate movements, everything should ultimately be strung together and done without pause, in one continuous dance-like sequence.

Depending on the rate at which you are breathing, the whole form should take between 5 and 8 minutes to complete, although more experienced tai chi enthusiasts will sometimes take longer. There are no hard-and-fast rules about speed – the most important thing is that you feel comfortable and relaxed.

The Short Yang Form: part 1

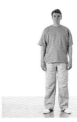
p42

p42

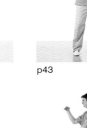
p43

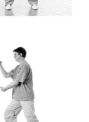
p43

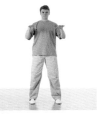
p44

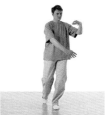
p44

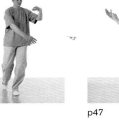
p45

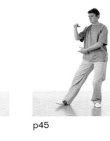
p45

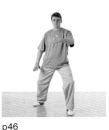
p46

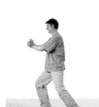
p46

p47

p47

p48

p48

p49

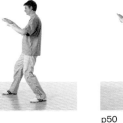
p50

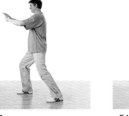
p50

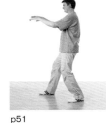
p51

p51

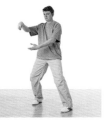
p52

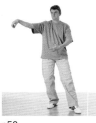

p52

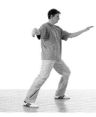

p53

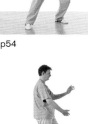

p53

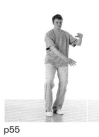

p55

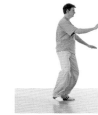

p54

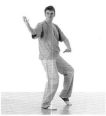

p54

p55

p56

p56

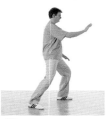

p57

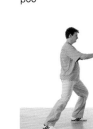

p57

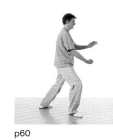

p58

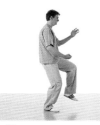

p58

p59

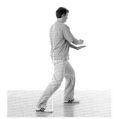

p59

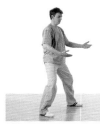

p60

p60

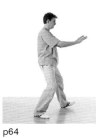

p61

p61

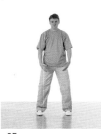

p62

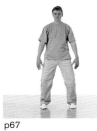

p62

p63

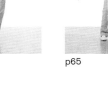

p64

p65

p65

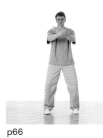

p66

p67

The Short Yang Form: part 2

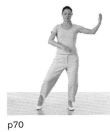
p70

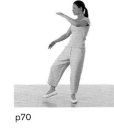
p70

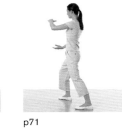
p71

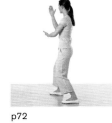
p72

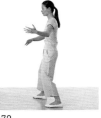
p72

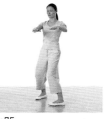
p73

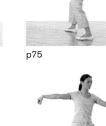
p74

p74

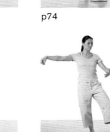
p75

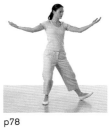
p75

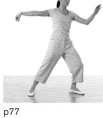
p76

p76

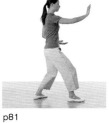
p77

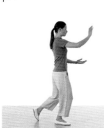
p77

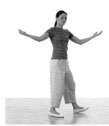
p78

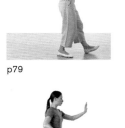
p79

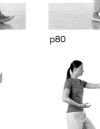
p79

p80

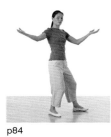
p80

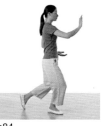
p81

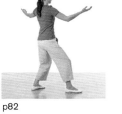
p82

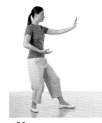
p82

p83

p84

p84

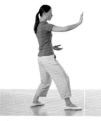 p85

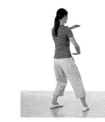 p86

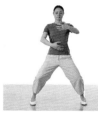 p86

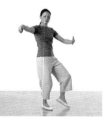 p87

 p87

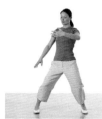 p88

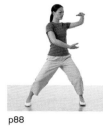 p88

 p89

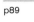 p90

 p90

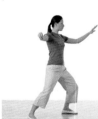 p91

 p92

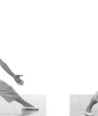 p92

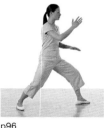 p92

 p93

 p93

 p94

 p95

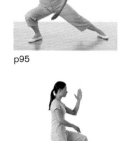 p95

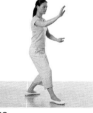 p96

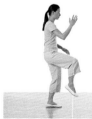 p96

 p97

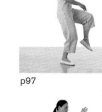 p97

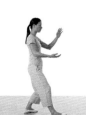 p98

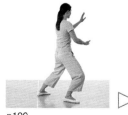 p98

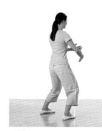 p99

 p99

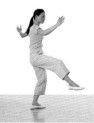 p99

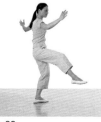 p100

 p100

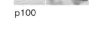

a summary of movements **137**

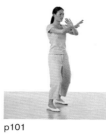 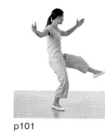 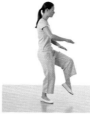 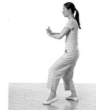 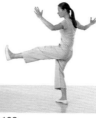

p101　　　　p101　　　　p102　　　　p102　　　　p103

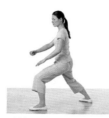 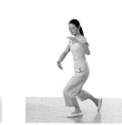 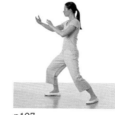 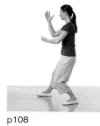 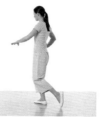

p104　　　　p104　　　　p105　　　　p105　　　　p106

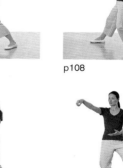 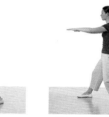 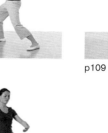 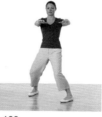 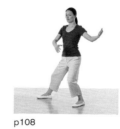

p106　　　　p107　　　　p107　　　　p108　　　　p108

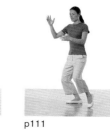 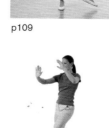 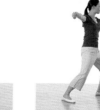 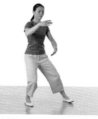 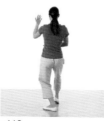

p108　　　　p108　　　　p108　　　　p109　　　　p109

p109　　　　p109　　　　p109　　　　p109　　　　p110

p110　　　　p111　　　　p111　　　　p112　　　　p112

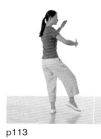

p113

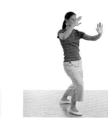

p113

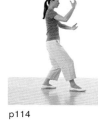

p114

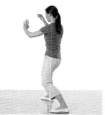

p114

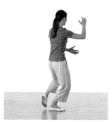

p115

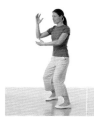

p115

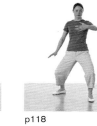

p116

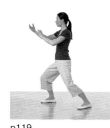

p116

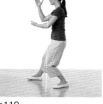

p117

p117

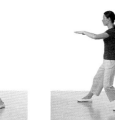

p118

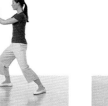

p118

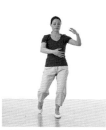

p119

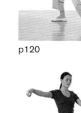

p119

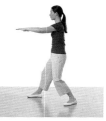

p119

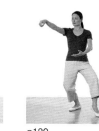

p119

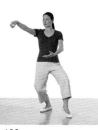

p119

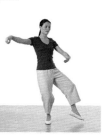

p120

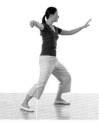

p120

p120

p120

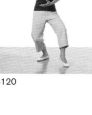

p120

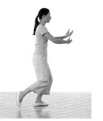

p120

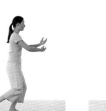

p120

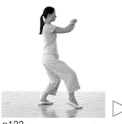

p120

p121

p121

p121

p122

p122

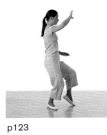 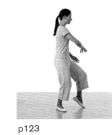 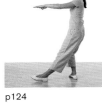 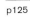 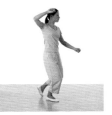

p123   p123   p124   p124   p125

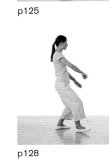 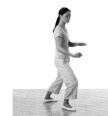 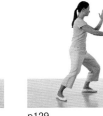 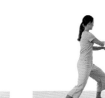 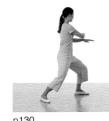

p125   p126   p126   p127   p127

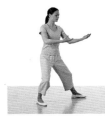 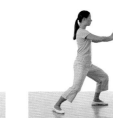 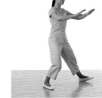 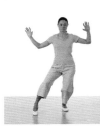 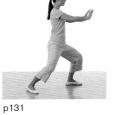

p128   p128   p129   p129   p130

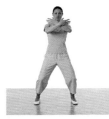 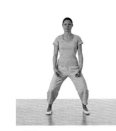

p130   p131   p132   p132   p133

p133   p133

Index

Acknowledgements

I would like to extend my thanks to everyone at Hamlyn who have helped in the production and design of this book. Special appreciation is also due to Jackie and Mark for undertaking the far from easy task of modelling for the tai chi form, and to Peter Pugh-Cook for his patience in taking the photographs with such sensitivity and skill. Thanks, too, Jenny and Neil for your kindness and support during the days of the photo-shoot, and for my partner Ruby who, as ever, provided the very best back-up and encouragement of all – and still managed to come out smiling!

Finally, if you have enjoyed this book, you might like to visit the author's web-site: www.orientalexercise.wanadoo.co.uk

Executive Editor Jane McIntosh
Project Editor Kate Tuckett
Executive Art Editor Leigh Jones
Designer Lisa Tai
Production Controller: Aileen O'Reilly
Special photography Peter Pugh-Cook
Models Jackie Chan, Mark Fletcher (www.yoga-taichi.com)

Picture Credits:
Special Photography: Peter Pugh-Cook
AKG, London/British Library 9; Alamy/John Foxx 27;
Bridgeman Art Library, London/New York 8; Corbis UK
Ltd/Wolfgang Kaehler 7